The Home Encyclopedia of

Symptoms, Ailments

and their

Natural Remedies

Carlson Wade

D0838954

PARKER PUBLISHING COMPANY
West Nyack, New York 10995

PARKER PUBLISHING COMPANY
West Nyack, New York

© 1991

This book is a reference work based on research by the author. The opinions expressed herein are not necessarily those of or endorsed by the publisher. The directions stated in this book are in no way to be considered as a substitute for consultation with a duly licensed doctor.

10 9 8 7 6 5 4 3 2 1

Library of Congress Cataloging-in-Publication Data

Wade, Carlson.
  The home encyclopedia of symptoms, ailments, and their natural remedies/Carlson Wade.
    p. cm.
  Includes index.
  ISBN 0–13–395492–7.—ISBN 0–13–395484–6 (pbk.)
  1. Medicine. Popular—Dictionaries.   I. Title.
RC81.A2W33   1991.
616.02′4—dc20   91–20632
                                                               CIP

ISBN   0-13-395492-7

ISBN   0-13-395484-6 (pbk.)

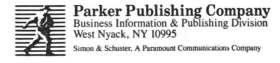
Parker Publishing Company
Business Information & Publishing Division
West Nyack, NY 10995
Simon & Schuster, A Paramount Communications Company

Printed in the United States of America

Dedication

To YOUR swift healing
and the Joy of Health
for your body and mind.

About the Author

Carlson Wade, one of the nation's foremost medical-nutrition reporte s, has written 26 books in the field of natural healing. He writes for many magazines, newspapers, and makes dozens of radio, television, and personal appearances every year. He is a columnist for the Nutrition and Dietary Consultant Journal, and hundreds of Mr. Wade's features and medical news columns have been published in countries world-wide, including France, Spain, Germany, and Japan. He is an accredited member of the American Medical Writers Association and the National Association of Science Writers.

OTHER BOOKS BY THE AUTHOR

Help Yourself With New Enzyme Catalyst Health Secrets

Inner Cleansing: How To Free Yourself From Joint-Muscle-Artery-Circulation Sludge

Eat Away Illness: How To Age-Proof Your Body With Anti-Oxidant Foods

Nutritional Healers: How To Eat Your Way To Better Health

How To Beat Arthritis With Immune Power Boosters

Immune Power Boosters: Your Key To Feeling Younger, Living Longer

Foreword

Welcome to one of the greatest collections of natural healing techniques. Here is a comprehensive one-volume encyclopedia of fast, safe and thoroughly effective shortcuts to soothing relief for many distress signals that could happen to any member of your family. To yourself, also!

Carlson Wade, a highly respected medical researcher and reporter has collected proven healing remedies from the world's most recognized health practitioners. These remedies are described in simple terms. They are easy to use, quick to promote healing. Complete with case histories, drawn from private files, the presentation is easy to read. The remedies offer fast-acting healings for your most annoying and persistent medical problems.

This book is especially valuable because it may well keep you out of the doctor's office. How many times have you felt an ache, or a painful discomfort, a stomach upset, an allergy response, a general complaint of weakness? You make an expensive visit to your doctor, who tells you it is a minor problem that can be cleared up with a simple home remedy! It was not an emergency after all . . . if only you had known in advance!

Thanks to Carlson Wade's book, you WILL know the meaning of your ailment and whether the symptoms can be healed right at home as many doctors recommend.

Without the use of drugs, you can:

- Clear up your skin blemishes in a jiffy
- Relieve nagging headaches with simple home remedies
- Loosen up those muscle kinks that are giving you shooting spasms of pain
- Cool off the inflammation of burning arthritis
- Clear up embarrassing candida albicans or yeast infection with nutritional programs
- Correct many personal "female problems" with better home care and easy-to-follow remedies
- Revitalize your digestive system so you are free of the trouble of constipation, colitis, diarrhea, etc.
- How to nip a fungus infection in the bud, before it spreads to cause more hurtful injury
- How to fight cancer with your knife and fork
- Boost your immune system

- Reduce your risk for cardiovascular distress
- And . . . much, much more!

When you have a health problem, you want fast relief . . . preferably without having to seek costly medical care. Carlson Wade's excellent volume covers just about every such problem—inside your body as well as outside—and taps the knowledge of many specialists to bring you quick remedies that might otherwise be costly in a hospital setting.

Carlson Wade's book will help you every day of your life. It is packed with beneficial remedies . . . right at your fingertips.

But there is more. Carlson Wade's Home Encyclopedia of Symptoms, Ailments, and Natural Remedies also features special help on the newest— and most effective—healing methods.

You'll find complete coverage of new treatments and procedures that speed up the process of healing. Look in the index to find the fast, proven medical answers you need for almost any disorder.

Using this book is the next best thing to being in a doctor's office. It is a landmark home guide for total wellness!

H. W. Holderby, M.D.

What this Book Will Do for You

It would be wonderful if you never became ill. Or hurt, never felt even a slight ache. You make every effort to build resistance to common and uncommon ailments. You select and prepare foods with the greatest of care, take regular exercise sessions, and use nutrients to boost your immune system.

So far, so good. You are practicing good health care and wise preventive medicine. And to a certain extent you will be rewarded with reasonably good health. But you live in the midst of a world of microorganisms waiting to penetrate your body to create disorders ranging from painful arthritis to breathing difficulties, from digestive disorders to premature aging, from hypertension to osteoporosis . . . and the risks go on and on. For example:

- Where did those skin blotches come from?
- Do those chest pains warn of a heart attack?
- Are stiff fingers a symptom of approaching arthritis?
- Why have you suddenly been troubled with embarrassing female disorders that refuse to go away?
- No matter what you eat, why do you have a "rebound" attack of gastro-intestinal distress?

Here is a book that describes in simple-to-follow, easy-to-read, everyday language the more than 100 all-too-familiar symptoms that can cause hurt, confinement, fear, and even disability, if not treated promptly. The natural remedies that help your body adjust speedily are clearly described. They use natural everyday items . . . many are probably in your pantry right now. Some of the healing remedies are absolutely free! And so easy to use, too!

This book was written to help everyone who is concerned about health (and who isn't?) and wants to have quick, at-a-glance descriptions of ailments, symptoms and the healing remedies. Even if you are not sick, you may not necessarily be enjoying the full benefits of total health. It may be that you are not yet showing any overt symptoms of illness. Why wait until you develop skin aging, painful shoulders and legs, chronic insomnia, osteoporosis, high blood pressure (the invisible killer that has no outward symptoms), cardiovascular pain, hardening of the arteries?

This book will provide clues to the slightest symptoms, so that you can take speedy efforts to nip the ailment in the bud. With a flip of the page, you discover what those symptoms mean, their causes, and how to find relief.

That pain in the neck hurts and makes you stiff; discover a simple exercise and water remedy that gives relief in a jiffy.

Troubled by irregularity but avoid laxatives because of side effects, read about simple foods that can make you regular almost overnight.

Allergies giving you a stuffy nose and watery eyes and making you feel miserable . . . make some changes in your living/working space and follow nutritional programs to overcome this sensitivity.

Skin aging too rapidly, making you old before your time . . . try certain foods and creams that erase wrinkles . . . discover how plain water helps you look "forever young" in days!

Digestive upset causing you painful spasms and reactions . . . nutritional remedies and food adjustments can rebuild your insides and free you from hurtful pains.

This book is a family encyclopedia dedicated to your improved and rejuvenated health. It offers drug-free remedies for hundreds of problems that are hurtfully interfering with your enjoyment of daily living.

It is an easy-to-use and a speedily effective source of drugless healing. It helps you avoid going to your doctor for every small complaint. Its purpose is to better acquaint you with your body, make you aware of signals that call for quick help and relief.

With the use of foods, specific nutrients, juices, herbs, hydrotherapy, fitness, and emotional remedies, you can free yourself from the hurt . . . quickly and safely.

This alternative method of "biological medicine" is the healing art of the future. You can restore health, free yourself from drugs and their side effects, prevent or avoid surgery, live longer and more happily. This book will show you how . . . turn the page!

Carlson Wade

Contents

H

I

J

K

L

M

O

P

R

S

T

U

V

W

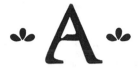

ACNE

Symptoms

Acne is a catchall term for a group of symptoms including pimples, black-heads, whiteheads, little or enlarged bumps and ridges on the skin. It is a condition caused by clogging of the skin pores. Acne develops when the level of *androgens* (male sex hormones) accelerates in the body at puberty, during which time there is a boosted outpouring of hormones in the testes and ovaries. This upsets the normal processes of the skin, causing the sebaceous glands (fat-producing glands at the root of the hair follicles) to speed up oil production. Ordinarily, these glands release a balanced amount of oil to maintain the skin at a proper level of lubrication. But when prodded by the androgens, the cells lining the hair follicles are manufactured at a very fast rate. These cells are discarded and tend to clump together with the oil. They clog the follicles and give rise to pimples, or acne.

Natural Remedies

Acne is not caused by particular foods, unless you have an allergic reaction to certain products. James E. Fulton, Jr., M.D., Ph.D., founder of the Acne Research Institute in Newport Beach, California, confirms this fact. "Chocolate does not cause acne. Dirty hair or skin does not cause it. Sex, either too much of it or a lack of it, does not cause it either."[1]

What then are the causes and what are some remedies? "Stress, sun exposure, seasonal changes and climate can precipitate an acne attack. Working women are especially vulnerable. They are prone to lots of stress, plus they tend to wear makeup a lot," says Dr. Fulton.

Makeup May Be to Blame. Certain products, in particular, may cause acne outbreaks. Dr. Fulton notes, "Oil-based makeup is the problem. The pigments in foundation makeups, rouges, cleansing creams, or night moisturers are not the problem; neither is the water in the products. It is just the oil. The oil is usually a derivative of fatty acids that are more potent than your own fatty acids. Use a non-oil based makeup if you are prone to acne."

1

Which Ingredients to Avoid? Cosmetic products that have lanolins, D and C red dyes, isopropyl myristate, laureth-4 and sodium lauryl sulfate should be avoided. They are too rich for your skin and could trigger an acne outbreak.

Quick Test for Cosmetic Safety. Dr. Fulton suggests you use a sheet of 25 percent cotton-bond typing paper. Rub a thick streak of your makeup onto it and put the paper in a cool place. After 24 hours, look for an oil ring. "Within a day, the oil will spread out. You should see the big grease ring. The bigger the ring, the more oil you have in your makeup. I urge you to keep away from makeup that produces big oil slicks."[1]

Hands Off Your Skin. Avoid irritating an already irritated skin. "Do not squeeze your pimples or whiteheads," cautions Peter E. Pochi, M.D., professor of dermatology at Boston University School of Medicine. "A pimple is an inflammation, and you could add to the inflammation by squeezing it and cause an infection. Normally, a pimple will last from one to four weeks, but it will always go away."

Which Pimple Can Be Squeezed? Dr. Pochi says that you can clear away one kind of pimple with the squeeze method. "Look to see if the pimple has a small central yellow pus head in it. If so, gentle squeezing usually pops these open rather nicely. Once the pus is out, the pimple will heal more rapidly."

Natural Remedy for Blackheads. Try the squeeze attack, too. "A blackhead is a very blocked pore. The material inside this blocked pore is solid, and the surface of the pore is widened," explains Dr. Pochi. "The black part of the blackhead is not dirt. Actually, we dermatologists are not certain what it is, but we do know that it will not erupt in a pimple." Squeeze gently, and you can ease the crop of blackheads.

Stress, Women, Acne. Stress may contribute to both hormonal upset and chronic adult acne in women, explains Dr. Pochi. "Stress can trigger an overproduction of adrenal male hormones in women. That, in turn, can produce persistent acne which can be associated with more serious problems such as polycystic ovarian disease.
     "I have found that women with treatment-resistant acne may have decreased estrogen levels coupled with an increase in pituitary hormone that stimulates male hormones from the ovary. A similar hormonal pattern is found in women who have polycystic ovarian disease. When pituitary hormones stimulate the adrenal gland, as they do when people experience stress, it produces excessive androgen, a male hormone. The androgen,

in turn, stimulates oil production and probably causes the acne flareups."

Dr. Pochi observes, "Past clinical studies indicate that the endocrine system is closely linked to the development of acne. If a woman has persistent acne that does not respond to the usual therapy, it is possible there are underlying hormonal abnormalities."[2] By using stress-reduction methods, there is a possibility for balancing hormonal release and easing acne flareup.

Do You Have A Skin Allergy? Food does not necessarily cause acne, but some foods may make it worse and cause an allergic outbreak. Try each potential troublemaker one at a time (chocolate, ice cream, nuts and peanut butter, cheeses, iodized salts, seafoods—especially lobster, shrimp, clams and oysters—pork and bacon, carbonated and alcoholic drinks, spicy foods, tomato sauces, cold cuts, potato chips, popcorn and pickles), and keep a record of when each was eaten. This helps spotlight a food that worsens acne in a specific situation.

CAUTION: If a food increases acne in two or three days, omit it from your diet. If the acne does not change, the food may be eaten. Some drugs such as barbiturates (sleeping pills), contraceptives and iodides, may worsen the acne. Some girls and young women may find the condition worsens before their menstrual period. Other conditions that may aggravate acne include jobs involving grease (working on a car or near a greasy stove), exam pressure, or the stress-related excitement of important social functions that cause additional perspiration.

Building Resistance to Acne with Improved Daily Methods. Useful tips about acne-avoiding and erasing are offered by Jerome Z. Litt, M.D., dermatologist with Case Western Reserve University of Medicine. "While there is no easy cure for acne, you can control it to lessen its severity and to prevent the pitting and scarring that arise from neglect and self-medication.

Natural Methods

"The key to acne therapy is to control the overactivity of the oil glands, shrink them if possible, and destroy the bacteria that are responsible for the infection. And the earlier you treat your acne, the better." Dr. Litt offers these acne-resisting natural remedies:

- Wash your face thoroughly at least three times daily.
- Don't pick or squeeze. This may aggravate the condition and lead to infection and scarring.
- Shampoo your hair frequently.

- Keep your hair off your face. Do not use hairsprays, mousses, or greasy hair dressings.
- Avoid greasy cosmetics.
- Avoid creamy suntan lotions.
- Facials are not recommended because the creams and lotions force more oil into the already clogged pores.
- If you have acne near your mouth, stop your fluoridated toothpaste for a few months and note whether it makes any difference.
- Avoid emotional stress. The chemicals released by your body during anxious and stressful situations stimulate the adrenal gland to produce more of the male-type hormone (more so in women!) which, in turn, stimulates the overproduction of skin oil.
- If your physician has prescribed tetracycline for your skin, do not take multiple vitamin supplements containing iron. Iron interferes with the absorption of tetracycline.[3]

Herbal Remedies. Relief is often obtained by using natural herbs. Dr. Jack Soltanoff, chiropractor-nutritionist and holistic healer of West Hurley, New York, suggests the following: "After washing or thorough gentle cleansing, rinse your skin with an infusion of chamomile, which is purifying, yarrow which helps eliminate toxins, catnip which is antiseptic, lavender which is cleansing and antiseptic, or thyme which is a strong germ killer. (These herbal infusions are available at many pharmacies and herbal outlets.)

"Dab pimples with undiluted lemon juice to kill germs, cool inflammation and improve circulation. Apply a calendula ointment to reduce inflammation and improve local healing. Acne may be relieved by changes in your dietary habits; check to see if you have allergic reactions. Many of my acne-prone patients find relief when they eliminate refined sugars, cut down on fats and dairy products."[4]

❧

CASE HISTORY—*From Spots To Smoothie With Natural Acne Remedies*

Recurring bouts of acne made Marsha J. so self-conscious, she isolated herself from others and faced the lonely potential of being a social outcast. Chemical preparations only worsened her crop of spots and caused unsightly breakouts. When someone called her "Spots" right to her blemished face, Marsha J. faced a choice: either remain in self-imposed isolation, or break free of the unsightly and stubborn acne.

She sought help from an herbal pharmacist who advised her to avoid eating excessively fatty foods (in her case, they led to skin outbreaks) and to use poultices of chamomile and yarrow on a twice-daily basis . . . in the morning and then shortly before retiring. The rinse would help purify and detoxify her skin. He also told Martha J. to carry a small bottle of undiluted lemon juice to apply over her skin at frequent intervals. Desperate for relief from the unsightly blemishes, Martha J. followed this program. She had doubts, claiming it was "too simple to be true." She was in for a welcome surprise. Within three weeks, the acne bumps and unsightly pimples started to subside. By the end of the fourth week, she saw herself in the mirror as having a smooth, soft and more youthful skin. She believed in the natural remedies now . . . and looked even happier when someone called her "Smoothie," while extending an invitation to a social function. Life would be beautiful . . . and so would Martha J.'s smooth skin!

ACQUIRED IMMUNE DEFICIENCY SYNDROME OR AIDS

Symptoms

AIDS is an acquired condition that causes a deficiency in the body's protective immune system and leads to a combination of illnesses (a syndrome.) AIDS is caused by the Human Immunodeficiency Virus (HIV). When HIV invades the immune system, the patient becomes unable to fight infections and tumors. The virus may also attack the brain. It may take anywhere from a few months to many years for the HIV-infected person to develop AIDS. The patient may feel fine for anywhere from a few weeks to several years after infection occurs. During this period, the immune system starts to make antibodies (special proteins that attack foreign substances) to try to fight the infection.

Some patients develop a generalized swelling of small glands in the neck, under the arms, in the groin and other areas. There may also be fever, weakness, diarrhea and weight loss. This set of conditions has been called the AIDS-Related Complex (ARC). Some patients die at the ARC stage, even before they develop AIDS. If the virus attacks the brain, the patient may become forgetful, apathetic, and unable to concentrate or perform routine tasks.

How is HIV spread? Live HIV is found in high concentrations in the infected person's blood and semen or vaginal secretions. For the disease to spread, one of these HIV-infected fluids must get *inside* a non-infected person's body. **DANGER:** That happens mainly through sexual contact or intravenous drug use in which needles and syringes are shared. (A smaller number of cases involve hemophiliacs and others who receive transfusions of HIV-infected blood, and babies born to HIV-infected mothers.) In the United States, most cases of AIDS involve homosexual men and intravenous drug users. However, sexually transmitted AIDS is spreading among bisexual men (men who have sex with both men and women) and among heterosexual men and women—often from sexual contact with intravenous drug users.

Basically, sex is the most common way of spreading AIDS. Exposure occurs when the blood or semen that contains the infected cells is passed into the bloodstream of an uninfected person. **DANGER:** If either partner has open sores on the sexual organs, HIV can pass from one body to the other more easily during intimacy.

Natural Remedies

The program involves several immune-boosting methods. You will help prevent AIDS if you

- Avoid sexual contact with intravenous drug users and their sexual partners.
- Avoid having multiple sexual partners. Avoid sexual contact with men and women who have multiple sexual partners, whether they are heterosexual or homosexual.
- Avoid sexual contact with anyone whose medical history and current state of health are unknown to you.
- Avoid sexual contact with people known or suspected of having AIDS (or other sexually transmitted diseases).
- Avoid any sexual contact without the use of physician-recommended condoms. And remember, choosing your sexual partner carefully is more important than relying on a condom.
- Do **NOT** inject illegal drugs. Just do **NOT!** If you inject drugs, never share needles or syringes. *Never . . .* not with anyone.
- To dispose of intravenous equipment, soak it in bleach, wrap it thickly in cloth or paper, and throw it away. Make certain no one can ever find it or get scratched by it.
- Whether or not you use drugs, *never* share a toothbrush, razor, or anything else that might have another person's blood on it.

Nutritional Remedies

"AIDS is a destructive syndrome," explains Myron Winick, M.D., of the Columbia University College of Physicians and Surgeons. "Malnutrition occurs because nutritional requirements increase. The intake and absorption of nutrients are impaired." Dr. Winick emphasizes that nutritional therapy does not necessarily cure AIDS, but the key is to better the lifestyle of the patient. He recommends a nutritional profile on a personal, per patient basis and "a multiple vitamin-mineral supplement taken daily that has 100 percent of the Recommended Daily Allowance."[5]

Glutamine—Amino Acid Remedy. Boost resistance with glutamine, suggests Richard J. Andrassy, M.D., of the University of Texas Health Science Center. "Glutamine is good for the mucosal lining of the body; it builds resistance to the symptoms." This amino acid is available as a supplement at many health food stores.

Arginine—Amino Acid Remedy. Dr. Andrassy explains, "Arginine helps heal wounds, increases the utilization of much-needed protein throughout the body and helps boost the immune system . . . these are all needed to stimulate the immune system." Many AIDS victims are deficient in these two amino acids. "You don't cure AIDS with these nutritional remedies, but you do make life more comfortable."[6]

Low-Fat Diet Is Helpful. Boost immunity to AIDS and also help control symptoms on a low-fat diet. Stimulate cell-mediated invigoration on less fat and less cholesterol—both of these substances may suppress immune function and could even increase the susceptibility to infection.[7]

Zinc Is Vital. Nutritional scientists note that nearly all AIDS victims show very low serum zinc levels. Promiscuous sexual behavior could create a risky zinc loss through the semen and prostate fluid that is expelled. The resultant low body-zinc level could depress immune abilities and make AIDS infection more likely in those who are exposed to the virus. Zinc is needed to help build immune bodies to fight AIDS and other infection. This mineral is able to detoxify harmful invading bacteria and viruses. Boost your immune system to ease AIDS with zinc.[8] About 150 milligrams of zinc daily is generally regarded as helpful as a natural remedy for a faltering immune system.

Nutritional Intervention. "We endorse the remedy of initiating nutrition support at the first sign of symptomatic HIV infection," advises Kassandra Rodriguez, M.D., Director of the AIDS Clinical Inpatient Unit at Jackson Memorial Hospital, in Miami, Florida. "Upon diagnosis, a registered dietician (RD) should be consulted. It is hypothesized that early nutrition intervention may prevent wasting (loss of lean body mass), enhance response to drug therapy, and improve the overall quality of life. The initiation of nutrition support may make the difference between a person who continues to function independently and one who is bedridden and totally dependent on others."[9]

ALCOHOLISM

Symptoms

Alcohol is the nation's number one drug problem, although many people do not think of the active ingredient in a drink as a drug. But the chemical compound called ethyl alcohol, often shortened to ethanol, is a mood-altering drug. It is not what you drink that causes the symptoms, but how much alcohol you consume.

Ethanol, present in all liquor, takes effect almost immediately. Unlike food, it does not have to be digested. It passes through the wall of the stomach and small intestine directly into the blood where it is carried to the brain.

Small amounts act as a stimulant and give the drinker a sense of well-being and relief from tension. As larger amounts are consumed, it acts as a depressant. That does not mean the drinker's mood becomes depressed or sad, although it might; the depressant effect acts on certain parts of the brain, impairing its ability to control various parts of the body. A wobbly walk and slurred speech are typical symptoms of over-drinking, although alcohol does not act directly on the legs or tongue. Instead, it depresses the part of the brain responsible for walking and talking.

More advanced symptoms include low blood sugar (hypoglycemia), dizziness, upset stomach, diarrhea, anemia, dehydration.

Natural Remedies

The first plan is to put limits on your drinking. Just as you have learned to control other influences on your diet, such as caffeine, cholesterol, sodium and sugar, you can control your desire to drink. For example:

1. Set your own limit based on alcohol's effect on your personal health and fitness goals. If you're going to a party or dinner

with friends, decide how much is too much ahead of time and stick to your limit.

2. Have something to eat. Even if you cannot eat a whole meal, eat something—especially a bit of fat. A glass of milk, for example. Never drink on an empty stomach!

3. Sip drinks, don't gulp. You'll still feel the effects, even as you stick to your own limit.

4. Dilute your drink. Given the choice between a tall diluted drink and a short potent drink, go for the tall one.

5. Do not drink to relieve symptoms. Alcohol is a depressant, and can actually exaggerate feelings of anxiety, pain or depression—not relieve them.

6. Don't drink to signals; e.g., lunchtime, quitting time, before dinner, nightcap, etc.

7. Don't drink and drive. Depending on your body weight, it takes about one hour to metabolize each drink. If you drink faster than one drink per hour, alcohol accumulates in your blood and can take longer to be metabolized.

8. Dilute drinks with water or fruit juice to slow absorption of alcohol. DANGER: Be wary of carbonated mixers and hot drinks, which are absorbed faster.

9. Nurse your drinks; you'll be less likely to over-imbibe. As a rule of thumb, limit yourself to one drink per hour. (That is how long it takes your body to metabolize the alcohol in one drink.) But no more than four drinks on any occasion. No more than seven drinks a week.

10. Be aware of the alcohol content of various drinks. About the same amount of alcohol is found in: 5 ounces of wine, 12 ounces of regular beer and 1 ½ ounces (one jigger) of 80-proof distilled spirits. DANGER: The alcohol in wine is more rapidly absorbed than that in beer or hard liquor.

11. Before you drink at a party, try high-protein foods that are low in salt to help slow alcohol absorption and control thirst. Try seafood, vegetables with dips made from beans, tofu, yogurt, cottage cheese; try chicken tidbits or small meatballs. Avoid salty snacks such as chips, commercial dips, smoked fish, cheese snacks. Salt increases drinking urge.

12. If you take two or more drinks a day, also take a multi-vitamin supplement containing the Recommended Daily Allowance (RDA) along with calcium and magnesium.

Nutritional Remedies

To build resistance to the urge for liquor and to help promote healing of the ravages of alcohol, rebuild your body with nutritional remedies.

Ornithine. An important amino acid that helps regenerate healthy liver tissue, much needed among heavy drinkers.

Cysteine. A sulfur-containing amino acid that has a remarkable ability to neutralize the damaging aldehydes (toxins) that occur from drinking. Cysteine also initiates the production of a toxin-mopping enzyme (glutathione) which helps wash out irritants from the system.

Glutamine. Nutritional scientist, Dr. Roger J. Williams has found that supplements of glutamine help alcoholics overcome their addiction. Glutamine is converted to gamma-aminobutyric acid (GABA), a most powerful chemical messenger in the brain that gives you stronger control over the urge to drink. About 6,000 milligrams of glutamine daily will help you break free from alcoholic addiction.[10]

Vitamin B Complex. Thiamine deficiency is common among drinkers because alcohol interferes with its absorption. Thiamine is needed because the body devours huge amounts in order to burn alcohol as a carbohydrate. Vitamin B_6 and Vitamin B_{12} are often low or absent in the drinker. Basically, B-complex absorption is reduced or impaired because alcohol changes bone marrow cells and serum iron levels creating a deficiency.

Vitamin A + Zinc = Natural Remedy for Alcoholism

Normally, the enzyme system alcohol dehydrogenase (ADH) functions to stimulate vitamin E to provide healthy vision. But in the drinker, ADH is involved with processing alcohol, thereby reducing its use for vision. One team of medical researchers has suggested that drinkers take vitamin A supplements even if deficiency symptoms are not yet visible.[11]

ADH contains zinc, which makes it an important mineral to be taken by the drinker, especially with Vitamin A. This combination helps the body metabolize ADH, minimizes the ravages of alcohol, and also promotes better self-control.

Vitamin E. In test studies, this vitamin helps control and minimize the harmful effects of toxins on the liver.[12]

Selenium. This mineral is needed to help guard against excessive organ damage from alcoholism, especially to the liver.

Choline. This vitamin of the B Complex is needed to inhibit or at least reduce fatty infiltration in the liver of drinkers.

Carnitine. A trace element, carnitine acts as a "fat shuttle," whereby it helps protect against harmful irritation, as seen in cirrhosis of the liver.

Rebuild your body and mind to overcome alcoholic addiction and free yourself from the life-threatening consequences of this drug!

ALLERGIES

Symptoms

Allergies are mistakes the body makes by overreacting to otherwise innocent substances. These may be taken into the body by being inhaled or swallowed, or by contact with the skin. Such sensitizing substances are called allergens. Examples of offenders include pollens, molds, house dust, animal danders (skin shed by dogs, cats, horses, rabbits), animal urine and saliva, feathers (as in feather pillows), kapok, wool, chemicals used in industry, foods, drugs, insect venom. Factors such as temperature extremes and sunlight can also trigger allergic reactions. Common allergy symptoms include a congested or runny nose, itching and tearing of the eyes, tightening of airways (leading to wheezing and shortness of breath), itching welts and other rashes of the skin; also stomach and bowel problems such as cramps, nausea, irregularity.

Natural Remedies

Help yourself overcome the assault of allergens with a set of 10 steps to minimize irritations:

1. Smooth, uncluttered, easily cleaned surfaces are helpful; bare floors and walls are suggested. Small objects, such as knick-knacks, books and records, should be placed in drawers or closed cabinets. Avoid making your bedroom a library.

2. If carpeting is unavoidable, use low pile types.

3. Place zippered, airtight plastic or fabric encasings on all pillows, mattresses and box springs.

4. Vacuum floors and wood furniture surfaces weekly. Remove chenille spreads, if present, and avoid stuffed items such as quilts

and comforters. Do not use feather or down pillows. Replace your synthetic pillows every two to three years.

5. If you must clean, a dust mask should be worn. These masks provide good protection and are re-usable.

6. In homes with forced air systems, central electrostatic precipitators or HEPA filters may reduce allergen levels; however, these expensive options are no substitute for effective dust-proofing measures within the home. Precipitators may generate irritating levels of ozone (pollutant in the environment) during prolonged operation, and all units require regular maintenance. Free-standing "filter" units have uncertain value. However, central fiberglass filters, replaced monthly, are considered helpful.

7. These anti-dust measures, along with dehumidifiers, help to minimize the growth of mites, microscopic insects found in house dust. Dehumidifiers are also useful in controlling the growth of molds in the home. Condensation on surfaces and seepage of ground water should be restricted. Avoid moldy firewood, hay and dried plants; keep jute and straw accessories dry. Clean up food spills immediately. For mold-sensitive people, boiler-type vaporizers at room level may be preferable if humidification is considered essential. Keep houseplants to a minimum, as they tend to promote mold growth.

8. Outdoors, leaf-raking, cutting grass, and hiking through dense undergrowth tend to worsen symptoms. A dust mask may make these activities more bearable. Elimination of ragweed and wild grasses as well as pollen-producing yard trees is also recommended.

9. Though central air conditioning is preferable, window units can be helpful, particularly in the bedroom. All doors and windows should be tightly shut. The window air conditioner (with its vent closed) should be operated only during room occupancy, preferably at night, when pollen levels are low.

10. Respiratory irritants to avoid: cigarette smoke, powders, such as laundry detergents and dry milk, shoe polish, cleaning products, and scented cosmetics. Either eliminate these items or confine them to well-ventilated areas.

Six Steps to Build Immunity to Allergies

To help boost your immune system so that you have greater resistance to allergies, try these six steps as part of your daily lifestyle (they are surprisingly easy and extremely effective as immune boosters):

1. Follow a regular exercise program. Physical activity helps open your passageways and protect against respiratory congestion.

2. Try to avoid outdoor activities too early in the day when pollen and mold counts are very high. Schedule activities for late afternoon or early evening.

3. If it is dry and windy outside, try to remain indoors.

4. Protect yourself from irritants, such as chlorine in pools and chemical sprays. They increase your sensitivity to inhaled allergens. If you must swim in a chlorinated pool, put on leak-proof goggles, nose clips, and ear plugs.

5. Indoors? Use an air-conditioner and keep windows closed.

6. Rinse your nasal passages with ordinary salt water. A refreshing allergy-fighting remedy can easily be made at home: mix ¼ teaspoon salt in one cup of lukewarm water. Then squirt the solution into your nose with a syringe.

CASE HISTORY—*Builds Immunity To "Hopeless" Allergies*

Ordinary yard work often sent Robert C. into a coughing, sputtering, choking allergic reaction. To worsen his situation, he had recurring allergy attacks on the job at a warehouse, which had dust, pollutants from incoming shipments, and constant temperature changes ranging from very cold to extremely hot in different sections of the complex. Robert C. took medications but they made him drowsy; his words came out slurred, and he had dry nasal passages that caused irritation. He sought help in order to cope with his "hopeless" allergies (and safeguard his job, too).

An environmentalist recommended the preceding ten-step program as well as the additional six-step immune-boosting remedies. Desperate, Robert C. followed them as much as possible. He took to wearing a dust mask, even if co-workers laughed and joked. Robert C. had the last laugh. Within two weeks, he could breathe comfortably even though he continued working under similar conditions as before. The protective methods had boosted his immune system, and he could breathe more easily, with fewer and fewer allergic attacks. Before the end of one month, he was so strengthened, he could look ahead to freedom from allergies . . . and yes, he did have the last hearty and refreshing laugh. Thanks to an invigorated immune system, he no longer needed medications!

———————————————— ❧ ————————————————

CASE HISTORY—*A Pinch of Salt Opens Choked Air Passageways*

Polly B. had infrequent bouts with allergies. She had a stuffed nose that sent her into panic because she could not breathe! Chemical medications offered some relief but gave her dizzy spells and irritated her respiratory tract. Polly B. explained the situation to a local naturopathic physician who suggested she try a simple natural remedy: whenever her allergic attack constricted her nasal passageways and she felt a choking sensation, she was to squirt the salt water solution into her nose with a syringe. "Carry a small bottle with a syringe wherever you go. If you develop an attack, head for the ladies' room and use the squirt. It works swiftly and has no side effects because it is natural," was the advice. Polly B. followed the program. No longer did she face medication aftereffects. Her choked air passageways opened in seconds with this simple natural remedy. She breathed with relief and said gratefully, "A pinch of salt has made me free of allergy attacks!"

ALZHEIMER'S DISEASE

Symptoms

First described by neurologist Alois Alzheimer in 1906 in the medical literature, it is a condition that produces intellectual impairment. It is characterized by the deterioration of the ability to think; it is a slow, progressive wasting of the brain. Alzheimer's will strike five percent of the population who reach 65, and more than 20 percent of those who reach 85. Gradually, the person becomes more forgetful, particularly about recent events. The individual may neglect to turn off the oven, misplace things, recheck to see if a task was just done, may take longer to complete a chore that was previously routine, may repeat already answered questions. As the disease progresses, memory loss increases. Other changes, such as confusion, irritability, restlessness and agitation are likely to appear in personality, mood and behavior. Judgment, concentration, orientation, and speech may also be affected. In the most severe cases, the disease may eventually render its victims totally incapable of caring for themselves.

Alzheimer's strikes at the heart of the brain's ability to integrate chemicals in the body by shutting off the production of vital neurotransmitters such as acetylcholine, serotonin, dopamine, GABA, noradrenalin and glutamate. These neurotransmitters are necessary for the maintenance of memory. Victims lose their "word-finding" ability; familiar words or expressions elude them. Familiar faces become strangers. Victims have difficulty finding their way around, forget where they put things, show impaired job performance and undergo personality changes—becoming inflexible, suspicious and hostile, for example.

The one definite diagnostic indicator of Alzheimer's is a pattern of brain-tissue plaques and tangles seen by microscope. Tangles are masses of fine filaments in the brain cells. These tangles run from a cell's nucleus to the axon, which functions like a cable to carry a cell's electrical impulses. Medical researchers suggest that these tangled filaments are brought about by the accumulation of aluminum in the body.

Natural Remedies

While Alzheimer's patients have unusually high levels of aluminum stored in certain areas of the brain (10 to 50 times normal levels), this buildup may or may not be a cause or a result of brain deterioration. The real question is how and when aluminum gets into the brain. To minimize this possible assault, plan to keep aluminum out of your body as much as possible. For starters:

Pre-treat Aluminum Cookware. Dr. Janet Greger, professor of nutritional science at the University of Wisconsin suggests, "To minimize the amount of aluminum that leaches from new aluminum cookware, follow this procedure. Wash the new pot or pan with hot sudsy water. Rinse. Then fill it up with water, boil it for two or three minutes and throw the water out. After that, there should be no need to worry about aluminum leaching into food." (You may want to avoid using aluminum cookware for safety's sake. Switch to glassware, stainless steel, or copper.)

Be Cautious About Medications. The largest source of aluminum is buffered aspirin and certain antacids. From these sources the total can range from 500 milligrams to 5000 milligrams in one day. "If you use antacids, you are getting a hundredfold, perhaps a thousandfold more aluminum from those products than from your food," says Dr. Greger.[13]

Be Cautious of These Aluminum Sources

Robert H. Garrison, Jr., a registered pharmacist in San Diego, California, points out, "Aluminum toxicity has been implicated in brain disorders associated with aging, such as Alzheimer's. Aluminum-injected rats learn at a slower rate and have aluminum concentrations in their brains parallel to those found in the brains of Alzheimer's patients." The pharmacist then lists these little-known sources of aluminum:

"Food additives (such as sodium aluminum phosphate used as an emulsifier in processed cheese), table salt (with added sodium silicoaluminate or aluminum calcium silicate) and potassium alum (used to whiten flour.) Acidic foods (such as rhubarb) cooked in aluminum pots leech the mineral into the water and available foods. Aluminum is also found in some antacids (as aluminum hydroxide gel) and some antiperspirants contain aluminum salts."[14]

Are You Cooking Aluminum? Since abnormal accumulation of aluminum is found in the brains of Alzheimer's patients, it is reasonable to suggest keeping intake to a minimum, if at all. You may be ingesting aluminum without knowing it. This is explained by food chemist A. Lione who points out that an aluminum coffee percolator is one such source. "The intake of aluminum has increased since the development of aluminum cookware, coffee pots, utensils and foil. The mineral in these cooking items dissolves into the food or beverage, increasing the aluminum content of a meal by several fold."[15]

Until more is known about the role of aluminum in the development and progression of Alzheimer's, it is wise to reduce intake of this metal by avoiding aluminum cookware and other aluminum-containing products.

Calcium Blocks Aluminum Absorption. Because the environment bombards us daily with aluminum, you may want to build resistance to its effects. Food scientist E. Somer suggests that adequate intake of calcium helps reduce aluminum absorption.[16]

Daily intake of 1,500 milligrams of calcium would appear to offer some appreciable protection against the invasion of unwelcome and crippling aluminum.

Choline: Will it Protect Against Memory Loss? It may help control the progress of memory loss . . . and perhaps it will build resistance or immunity to Alzheimer's. Scientists G. Rosenberg and K. Davis have reported on the use of choline for this condition. Choline is a nonessential nutrient produced in the body and supplied in the diet as a component of lecithin (phosphatidylcholine.) It is a constituent of acetylcholine, the neurotransmitter that is deficient in Alzheimer's. Drs. Rosenberg and Davis have found that supplementation with choline or purified soya lecithin (containing 90 percent phosphatidylcholine) on some occasions did slow the progression of memory loss in some patients. In some other tests, there was little effect on neurotransmitter levels or memory.[17] If choline or lecithin are useful, they probably are most helpful in the early stages of short-term memory loss.

Lecithin on a Daily Basis? Lecithin is a soya or sunflower food available in tablets or granules at most health food stores and major food outlets. It would be wise to take it on a daily basis to boost choline content. A simple remedy is to add two or three heaping tablespoons of lecithin granules to a whole grain breakfast cereal. This simple and tasty remedy may well help build resistance to Alzheimer's. Remember . . . one characteristic of Alzheimer's is the reduced ability of the brain to produce acetylcholine, the neurotransmitter in the brain responsible for memory. And lecithin is a rich concentrated source of choline that boosts production of this memory transmitter.

Natural Remedies to Help Improve Lifestyle

You need to encourage the person to function at the highest level possible. The following remedies are helpful:

- Avoid making any schedule changes that are not absolutely necessary. A routine is helpful. Frequently reassure the person of the surroundings and your concern for his or her well-being.
- The confused and disoriented person functions better in a dependable environment. Change can be upsetting. Try to minimize changing whatever is familiar.
- The person with dementia is especially sensitive to the moods and emotions of those in the immediate surroundings. Follow a calm approach. Be patient and understanding. Create an environment of safety and security.
- The Alzheimer's person cannot depend on his senses to be sure of well-being. Tell him and show him that he is safe and being cared for. The person does understand feelings and emotions, via non-verbal communication, even if he can no longer understand the spoken word. Your touch or smile fosters a sense of much-needed security.
- The Alzheimer's person has difficulty making sense of the environment. Frequent eye contact provides some stability and security.
- Your tone of voice and the words you use can demonstrate your respect for the person and your acceptance of him. CAREFUL: An angry or hostile tone adds to fear and confusion.
- Communicate by expressing one idea at a time. Use simple sen-

tences that require the interpretation of only one thought; these will be easier to remember and to respond to in kind.

- One way to deal with inappropriate behavior is to distract the person with another activity. Once distracted, he will likely forget what was disturbing him.

- Be punctual. Keep the time he waits to a minimum. His confusion and disorientation will increase if you keep him waiting in any unfamiliar environment. He may not understand or he may forget why he is waiting. He may become anxious and wander off.

- Keep in mind that the person mirrors the emotional state around him. If you are tense, grouchy and hurried, the patient will react this way.

- Speak in a clear, low-pitched voice. Use short, simple words, questions, sentences, and wait for a response before you continue. No response? Repeat your statement in exactly the same word order, without adding new words or explanations.

- If possible, demonstrate what you mean—gesture toward the street you want to walk toward, for example. Or show how a jacket or sweater should be put on. Do not argue!

- As a safeguard, some families sew name and address labels in clothing, as a precaution should the person wander off.

While the causes are being researched, it is known that the victims have tangled clumps of nerve fibers and patches of disintegrated nerve-cell branches in their brains. Also, a serious head injury could bring on a dimentia disorder. And, in persons with Alzheimer's disease, aluminum is found in the brain . . . but there is dispute over how it gets there and its effect on the brain. To help build resistance to this debilitating thief of life, it would be wise to minimize aluminum intake, boost lecithin-choline on a daily basis, keep active (mentally and physically). And . . . be kind to those who become victims of this disease.

ANEMIA

Symptoms

Anemia is a blood condition in which the number and/or size of red blood cells is altered. Because red blood cells transport oxygen from the lungs to the tissues, a reduction in their size or number reduces capacity (called the blood's oxygen-carrying capacity) to oxygenate the tissues. The red blood cells have an average life span of 120 days. Some cells must be replaced within three or four days. They require essential nutrients which include protein, copper, iron, folic acid, vitamins B_{12} and C, among others. If improperly nourished, the cells die and anemia may occur. Symptoms include lethargy, weakness, poor concentration, shortness of breath after minor physical effort, pale complexion, vulnerability to colds and infection, and mild depression. **DANGER:** In advanced stages of anemia, the fingernails become flat and thin, the tongue becomes smooth and waxy. Stomach disorders develop.

Natural Remedies

The most essential nutrient is that of iron. This mineral will help your body keep up a steady manufacture of new red blood cells packed with hemoglobin, the red-cell protein that moves oxygen throughout your body. **CAUTION:** Even mild anemia is an indication of iron deficiency; your body will drain out its store of iron until it is unable to have any more, then it cuts back on blood formation. This means you may be iron-deficient without being anemic. Here is an assortment of natural remedies to help your body build a rich, red bloodstream:

Iron in Lean Meats. The iron in meat is *not* in the fat so you may eat modest portions of lean, red meat for good amounts of iron. How much? About 3½ ounces daily (about the size of a deck of cards!) will be good for your bloodstream. You may also enjoy chicken and fish (much lower in saturated fat than meat) for iron.

Meat-Source Iron More Preferable. For the anemic person, meat may be preferable because it has the type of iron more useful to your needs. "Dietary iron occurs in two forms, *heme* and *non-heme,*" explains Marvin Adner, M.D., director of hematology at Framingham Union Hospital in Massachusetts. "Putting it simply, heme iron is the type that forms hemoglobin; it is available only from animal sources and is quickly metabolized by your body. Non-heme iron is the type available in plants and not all that easily absorbed.[18]

Limit Iron-Calcium Combination. In the presence of much calcium and phosphate, iron may be blocked from assimilation. You may continue enjoying much-needed calcium, but it would be best not to combine it with any iron-containing food at the same time. **TIP:** Do not take iron and calcium supplements together, since the calcium will bind with the iron, greatly reducing their iron absorption. If you must take both of these minerals, take them at different times of the day.

Enjoy Iron-Rich Plant Foods. You may build a rich and youthful bloodstream with minimal meat (if you so prefer) and more plant foods. Dried beans and peas (legumes) may have non-heme iron, but they should be included often. Other good sources include wheat bran, brewer's yeast, soybeans, prune juice. **TIP:** Iron absorption from vegetable foods is increased when a small amount of iron-rich animal food is eaten with it.

Cast Iron Cookware. A great way to help increase the iron content of your foods. Consider using cast iron pots for cooking. When cooked in iron pots, the iron content of long-cooking acidic foods, such as tomato sauce, will increase considerably. The iron content of breakfast cereals, brown rice casserole, and gravy and soups more than doubles when cooked in an iron pot. **TIP:** Iron can be water soluble. Use a cooking method that minimizes losses—steam or cook vegetables in small amounts of water, for the shortest possible time. Always use salt-free vegetable stocks for soups, casseroles and gravies.

Vitamin C + Iron = Rich Bloodstream. Vitamin C improves the absorption of non-heme iron in fruits, vegetables and whole grain fortified cereals. **TIP:** A glass of orange or grapefruit juice with your breakfast more than doubles the amount of iron your body absorbs. This happens mostly when you combine the Vitamin C foods *with* the iron foods. They work when eaten together!

Fiber: Too Much Can Rob Your Body of Iron. While dietary fiber is needed to keep cholesterol under control, too much will block non-heme iron absorption. (Some types of fiber, such as bran, latch onto non-heme iron and speed it through your digestive system so quickly, the iron has little chance for absorption.) **TIP:** Keep daily fiber intake to about 30 grams and your body will have full absorption of iron.

CAREFUL: Coffee or Tea Block Iron Absorption. If you drink these beverages *with* your meals, their tannins will latch onto iron, reducing its availability. **CAUTION:** A cup of tea with breakfast can block 75 percent of the iron that is not absorbed and you become shortchanged. **TIP:** If you must have a beverage at mealtime, select coffee substitutes or herbal teas that are free of caffeine and/or tannins.

Iron-Fortified Foods Are Great Blood Builders. Read package labels, especially on enriched breakfast cereals, and note iron content. **CAREFUL:** Not all are assimilated. If the label says "iron," it could be a compound beginning with "ferric" such as "ferric pyrophosphate," which is not easily or thoroughly absorbed. Instead, favor "ferrous sulfate," or "electrolytic iron," or an elemental iron, or "reduced iron." *Bonus:* If the iron-fortified food also has vitamin C, it will help you absorb the nutrients all the better. Be sure to read labels!

What About Supplements? If you are a young woman, especially if you are dieting, pregnant or otherwise undergoing changes, you should evaluate your diet and determine if you will benefit from supplements. TIP: If you take a supplement, do so at night on an empty stomach together with some orange juice. This promotes maximum absorption.

Blood-Building Iron Tonic. To a glass of orange juice, add one teaspoon brewer's yeast, one teaspoon thyme. Blend thoroughly and then drink. Best about two hours before bedtime, preferably on an empty stomach. *Benefit:* The Vitamin C from the orange juice will combine with the iron of the other ingredients to work swiftly for maximum absorption to enrich your bloodstream. Drink one glass every night as a great blood-building tonic. Tasty, too.

Nutritional Remedies

Folic Acid. Needed for normal formation of red blood cells. If there is a deficiency, you may face faulty cell division in which there are large, misshapen edges incapable of transporting oxygen. Found in whole grain breads and cereals, brewer's yeast, cooked asparagus, cooked beets, Brussels sprouts, and cantaloupe.

Vitamin B_{12}. Nourishes and improves health of your blood cells. It is found largely in foods of animal origin. Plants do not easily synthesize vitamin B_{12} (except for the leafy green vegetable, comfrey.) This vitamin is destroyed by heat and light. It is also available as a supplement.

Blood-Building Vitamin E. This is an important vitamin, needed to protect the red blood cells once they are formed. Vitamin E is an antioxidant, in that it protects red blood cell membranes from destruction by harmful molecules or free radicals. If you are deficient in Vitamin E, you run the risk of hemolytic anemia.
"The life of the flesh is in the blood," said the ancients. It is all too true in our modern times. Enjoy a more energetic quality of life with a youthful, enriched and well-nourished bloodstream!

CASE HISTORY—*Rebuilds Her Bloodstream While She Sleeps*

Troubled with bouts of anemia, Theresa L. was always feeling cold. She dozed off in the middle of an important sales meeting, much to her embarrassment and at the risk of her position as a marketing researcher. Theresa L. was always catching cold, felt weak, and was subject to bouts of depression. She wondered if she was "getting old," when she was only in her middle 40's. What was wrong? The answer came from her neighborhood cosmetician who did her fingernails and remarked how they looked so flat and thin, even pale. The beauty expert recognized the signs of anemia, having seen it in other customers. She urged Theresa L. to visit a local hematologist (blood specialist), who had helped other people. That was when Theresa L. found out she was anemic. The specialist recommended switching to iron cookware, combining Vitamin C foods with iron foods, then prescribed the aforementioned blood-building iron tonic. Results? Within two weeks, she had a youthful bloodstream. She was wide awake, no longer troubled by colds, energetic and youthful, with a cheerful disposition. Theresa L. said much could be traced to this tonic. She joshed that she could rebuild her bloodstream while she slept . . . with this tonic!

ANGINA PECTORIS

Symptoms

A heart attack is not the only result of cardiovascular illness. Another consequence of coronary heart disease is the chest pain called angina pectoris. When this occurs, open (but narrowed) arteries cannot deliver all the oxygen the heart needs. Angina pectoris can occur when the blood circulation to the heart is sufficient to meet normal heart needs, but inadequate when the heart's needs are increased, such as during physical exertion or emotional excitement. *Example:* Running to catch a bus could trigger an attack of angina . . . but walking to a bus stop would not. In this condition, there is pain in the chest and often in the left arm and shoulder. Another warning symptom is angina pain that lasts for more than 15 to 20 minutes. Typically, you may feel the pain as a pressing or squeezing sensation that starts in the center of your chest and moves to your shoulders or arms—usually along the left side— or even to your back, neck or jaw. The condition is often triggered by excessive physical and/or emotional stress, exposure to the cold or any situation that increases your heart's workload and demand for oxygen. Angina typically occurs because the coronary artery is blocked with so much "sludge" that the blood flow and its life-giving oxygen become reduced to less than 40 percent of normal. When blood flow and oxygen are restored within 10 to 15 minutes, the pain disappears.

Natural Remedies

Begin with a good attitude and a sincere desire to reshape your lifestyle for a healthier heart . . . and longer life. Help free yourself from angina pectoris with these heart-saving remedies.

Stop Choking Your Heart. Smoking will constrict your heart and lead to angina pectoris, among other hazards. Give up smoking . . . and stay away from "second stream" smoke . . . that is, from others who puff and blow smoke into your face, your lungs and your heart! Smoke causes a buildup of blood levels of carbon monoxide, which displaces oxygen. Since angina is triggered by an artery-choked heart begging for oxygen, smoking is an unequalled threat. Another danger is that cigarette smoke (from your tobacco or from others in your immediate vicinity) will cause your blood platelets to stick together, further choking your partially choked arteries. Researchers have learned that angina patients who give up smoking have one-half the fatality rate of those who have this heart-killing habit.

Control Fat Intake. One excessively fatty and salty meal can trigger an angina attack because it causes your blood pressure to shoot up suddenly. The danger is plaque, an artery-clogging mass of fat, cholesterol, blood-clotting substances, and cellular waste. Plaque builds up, choking arteries and blood flow. Angina, or chest pain, indicates its presence. Your arteries may become plastered with plaque because of fatty deposits that cling to artery walls. To avoid and/or reverse the condition, plan to cut back as much as possible on foods containing saturated fat (the kind that hardens at room temperature) and cholesterol. The American Heart Association recommends a diet containing less than 30 percent of calories from fat.[19]

- Eat no more than 3½ ounces of meat, poultry daily . . . about the size of a deck of cards.
- Meat should be lean, fat-trimmed before you cook, and fat-trimmed after you cook. Remove poultry skin before cooking. If you dislike the dryness that results, remove the skin before eating, instead.
- Keep *all* oils to a minimum of about 4 teaspoons daily. And use only monounsaturated or polyunsaturated oils.
- Best to avoid cholesterol-rich organ meats such as kidney, liver, and heart.

- Eat non-fat (or one percent fat) dairy products. Cheese? Favor those that are low-fat and *also* low-salt!

- Boost intake of fresh fruits and vegetables and whole grains. Oat bran is especially desirable in helping to bring down cholesterol-fat levels.

Omega-3 Fatty Acids. Researchers at the Mayo Clinic have found that the omega-3 fatty acids in fish oil may encourage relaxation of the coronary arteries. These natural substances ease spasms in coronary arteries clogged by atherosclerosis responsible for angina. The omega-3 fatty acids promote a "relaxing factor" that keeps the artery linings calm and smooth. Boost your intake of fish to help increase a supply of mega-3 fatty acids to counteract angina pain.[20]

Breathe Away the Pain. It may not be angina but hyperventilation. To reduce chest pain, train yourself to breathe properly. To avoid hyperventilation, get into the habit of breathing through your nose, not your mouth, and from your stomach, not your chest.

Tilt Your Body. If you have angina pain attacks at night, tilt the head of your bed up three or four inches. *Benefit:* Sleeping in this tilted position makes more blood pool in your legs; less goes to your heart's narrowed arteries. This may help cut down on your dependence upon nitroglycerine.

Feet on the Floor. If you are troubled with recurring angina attacks at night, before you habitually reach for your medication, change your position. Sit on the edge of your bed. Put your feet on the floor. If symptoms do not go away quickly enough, then continue with your medication.

Easy Does It. Stress can cause a sudden choking sensation and bring on an angina attack. You may try meditation, relaxation exercises or a brisk walk to help ease any stress situations. Resolve your conflicts in a peaceful way. It will help save your heart from angina attacks.

CASE HISTORY—*Overcomes Crippling Angina Pain With Nutritional Make Over*

Each recurring angina pain worsened until Anthony D. felt as if his heart was "tied up in a choking knot," and he feared hospitalization. Medications eased symptoms, but he did not want lifetime addiction to drugs and their side effects. His cardiologist outlined a fat-controlled food program, which offered welcome help. Increasing his consumption of fish and taking fish oil supplements helped Anthony D. overcome the crippling pain to the point where his doctor took him off medications and gave him a new lease on life. Anthony D. was known to say, "I've been made over into a new person with the help of nutrition. My heart does have nine lives!"

ARTHRITIS

Symptoms

The word arthritis literally means joint inflammation (*arth* = joint, *itis* = inflammation) and refers to more than 100 different conditions. Basically, there are two major forms of arthritis: (1) *rheumatoid arthritis* is an autoimmune disease involving chronic inflammation. The inflammation begins in the synovial membrane of the joints and spreads to other joint tissues. Eventually, outgrowths of the inflamed tissue may invade and damage the cartilage in the joints. This damage may change the shape of the joints, causing them to become deformed. (2) osteoarthritis involves the breakdown of cartilage and other joint tissues. Unlike rheumatoid arthritis, this form has little or no inflammation and does not affect the whole body. Symptoms usually begin slowly and may not seem important. One or two joints may ache or feel mildly sore, especially with movement. There may be constant nagging pain. The joints most commonly affected are the fingers, hips, knees and spine. It often appears in only one or two joints and does not spread further.

Basic Warning Signs

- Swelling in one or more joints
- Early morning stiffness
- Recurring pain or tenderness in any joint
- Inability to move a joint normally
- Obvious redness and warmth in a joint
- Unexplained weight loss, fever, or weakness combined with joint pain
- Symptoms such as these that last for more than two weeks

You should be aware of the warning signs of arthritis and see your health practitioner if they appear.

Natural Remedies

To help ease the ache and send arthritis into remission, rebuild your immune system and boost your resistance to this crippling ailment. Start today!

Shed Excess Weight. By getting rid of heavy poundage, you ease the stress and pain you feel in your spinal column, knees, hips, ankles and feet. Lighten the burden on your cartilage, removing the pressure on your bones and thereby reducing, and even eliminating, the incidence of swelling, inflammation, and pain.

Apply Heat and Cold. Both can be helpful. Heat can temporarily relax muscles and is especially helpful before exercising. You can apply heat to all the joints at once with a warm tub bath. To avoid fatigue, though, you should not stay in a warm bath for more than twenty minutes.

For warming and relieving individual joints, hot compresses can also be effective. Soak a towel in hot water, wring it out and place it on the painful joint. If you use a heating pad, keep it at a low heat setting and apply to the joint for a short period of time. Never lie on a heating pad or go to sleep with one left on your body.

For the temporary relief of pain and soreness, cold compresses can be applied to individual joints. An ice bag or ice cubes, or a small can of frozen juice placed in a plastic bag and wrapped in a towel offer the easiest kind of cold compress.

Do It Yourself Herbal Massage. Eucalyptus ointment (available at health stores and pharmacies) imparts soothing comfort beneath your skin surface to ease pain. Rub the ointment on the painful area and surrounding area. Then wrap the joint in plastic wrap. You'll feel a warmth that is most comforting. You may also apply moist heat with warm towels wrapped around the affected area. Eucalyptus is a most comforting herb that helps ease aches and pains of arthritis.

Ice That Pain Away. If you have stressed or overworked a joint and feel spasms of shooting pain, try an ice remedy. Put ice in a plastic bag, or else try a bag of frozen vegetables on the site of the pain. Let it remain for 15 minutes. Remove. Then repeat after waiting 15 minutes. Continue doing this until the pain has subsided . . . and next time, don't strain that joint! (If joints become hot, swollen or tender, use heat. Cold would make them painful!)

Willow Bark: Natural Aspirin. To ease pain, reach for the willow bark herb instead of a chemical aspirin. "In the long run, the most beneficial herb probably is willow bark," says Varro E. Tyler, Ph.D., Professor of Pharmacognosy at Purdue University. "That's simply because it contains *salicin,* which is similar to aspirin. But to treat arthritis properly, you would need a lot of bark." Willow bark is available at most health stores and herbal pharmacies.[21]

Vitamin C Builds Collagen and Cartilage. Rheumatoid arthritis patients are often deficient in vitamin C. With adequate amounts daily, ranging up to 1,500 milligrams, arthritis may be sent into remission. This nutrient helps regenerate much needed collagen and cartilage to minimize the effects of deterioration.

Fish Oils Cool Off Pain. The fatty acid in fish oils called eicosapentaenoic acid (EPA) is an effective adjunct therapy in the treatment of rheumatoid arthritis. Richard I. Sperling, M.D., a medical instructor at Harvard Medical School, found that patients who took fish oil capsules on a regular basis had fewer symptoms, and their morning stiffness improved. EPA or omega-3 fatty acids found in fish oils inhibit the production of certain leukotriene and prostaglandin substances. (These are responsible for inflammation and pain of the joints, as in rheumatoid arthritis.) Omega-3 fatty acids of fish oils "defuse" the hurt caused by the leukotriene and prostaglandin substances, and may promote amelioration of arthritis activity.[22] A rule of thumb, based on research, would suggest taking about 1.8 grams of EPA daily.

Avoid Excessive Fat. Oil-containing products such as margarines, fried foods, and salad dressings contain omega-6 fatty acids, another form of the substance that is not too desirable. **CAUTION:** Omega-6 fatty acids often cause inflammation in those who have rheumatoid arthritis. It would be best to minimize oil intake. Two oils that are exceptionally low in omega-6 fatty acids are olive oil and canola oil and are good substitutes for other oils. But keep these oils to a minimum, too. You need less fat!

------------------------------ ❧ ------------------------------

CASE HISTORY—*Nutritional Therapy Sends Arthritis Into Remission*

Agonizing pains, especially in the morning, forced Wilbur N. to cry out with pain. He needed help to climb out of bed, and each step was excruciating. He took prescribed medication which masked the pain, but he experienced diarrhea, stomach upset, and dizziness to the extent that he feared being turned into an invalid. He could hardly get to work. Was he facing a lifetime of helplessness? The answer came from an osteopathic physician who specialized in arthritic conditions. He prescribed a fitness program for Wilbur N., helped him shed excess weight, then boosted his intake of vitamin C and fish oils. He also suggested using willow bark as an herbal substitute for aspirin. Gradually, the pains subsided. If Wilbur N. cheated and neglected his nutrients, the pain came back with a vengeance, especially in the morning. He learned his lesson the hard way. He followed the nutritional and home healing programs very faithfully . . . and was rewarded with flexible joints, pain-free arms and legs, and a "get-up-and-go" vitality in the morning. His osteopathic physician pronounced the arthritis in remission . . . and Wilbur N. was able to work and live . . . independently!

ASTHMA

Symptoms

Asthma is a non-contagious disease of the lungs in which there is difficulty in breathing because of obstruction to the flow of air in the bronchial tubes. This obstruction is caused by swelling of the membranes lining the bronchial tubes, contraction of the surrounding musculature and a plugging of the tubes by thick mucus. The rush of air through the narrowed tubes produces wheezing—the noisy, whistling sounds that are typical of asthma. Episodes of asthma may last for a few hours, days, or even weeks. In severe attacks, breathing becomes increasingly difficult as the chest distends, and you need to use more and more energy just to breathe. Eating or talking may be too much of an effort, and the distress may be worsened by such simple things as laughing or lying down. Asthma may be present in less typical ways, such as a persistent, irritable cough or shortness of breath without apparent wheezing. A major cause of asthma is a sensitivity to certain non-living substances called allergens. Asthmatics become sensitive or allergic to these substances, which are ordinarily harmless to others. These sensitizing substances enter the body by being inhaled or swallowed.

Natural Remedies

Initially, you can minimize your discomfort by trying to avoid the worst-known irritants as much as possible. For example—

- Keep away from grassy fields, weedy lots, and similar areas, especially in the spring and fall.
- Avoid lawn mowing.
- Avoid exposure to fertilizers and insecticides.
- Stay away from dusty, smoky or polluted areas, and places full of chemicals or irritating fumes.
- Do not visit farms or zoos, or live near them, if you can help it.
- On days when the weather report announces high levels of pollen and mold spores, try not to go out until evening, when the count is lower.
- Do not use feather pillows, wool blankets, mattresses with jute or hair stuffing.
- Eliminate carpets, upholstered furniture, heavy draperies, and dust-collectors from your bedroom. When refurnishing your home, choose smooth, synthetic fabrics, simple wood or plastic surfaces for floors and furniture.
- Dust cloths, brooms and mops should be dampened before use, so that irritants are not scattered into the air. Try to stay out of a room where house cleaning is going on. If you must do a dusty household job, wear a surgical mask.
- No dogs, cats, or other hairy animals in your home—no birds, either. If you must keep a pet, by all means keep it out of your bedroom.
- Be alert to changing weather conditions, including changes in temperature, humidity, barometric pressure, and strong winds. All are likely to affect and irritate airways.

Relax to Breathe More Easily. If you have an asthma episode, you are short of breath. You feel nervous and breathe faster. More air is trapped in your lungs. You feel increasingly worse if pollution levels are high. *Note:* Before you can breathe in fresh air, you need to get the stale air out; that's hard if your airways are clogged and narrowed. Do **NOT** gasp for air. Instead, follow these steps:

1. Relax. Let your neck and shoulders droop.
2. Breathe in slowly through your nose.
3. Purse your lips in a whistling position, and blow out slowly and evenly, taking twice as long as you did breathing in.
4. Relax. Repeat the pursed-lip breathing, until you no longer feel breathless. If you get dizzy, rest for a few breaths.

When you breathe out slowly through pursed lips, you keep up the air pressure in your airways. That helps them stay open so that you can breathe out more stale air, and return your breathing to normal faster. Once you've gained control of your breathing, maintain control by staying relaxed and breathing slowly.

Keep Away from Food Additives. In particular, metabisulfite and monosodium glutamate (MSG) can trigger an asthmatic attack. Most commonly, metabisulfite is found in beer, wine, shrimp, and chemically-dried fruits, especially apricots. CAREFUL: Sulfites may be used as a "freshener" upon fruits and vegetables, especially in salad bars, to keep them looking fresh. MSG may also bring on an attack. Because it is commonly used in Oriental foods, it is known as the "Chinese Restaurant Syndrome." It would be best to avoid foods containing such additives.

Vitamin B_6 Builds Immunity to Asthma. Researchers at the University of Texas have found that those who develop MSG-induced attacks are also deficient in vitamin B_6. They noted that when a sensitive patient would take 50 milligrams daily of Vitamin B_6, there was greater resistance to such reactions. MSG seeks a weak link in your immune system to penetrate and provoke an asthmatic attack. It is vitamin B_6 that seems to be able to protect and boost the immune system to help resist reactions.[23]

Reduce Frequency of Asthma with Vitamin B_6. Another research team noted that a group of asthma patients had marked deficiencies of vitamin B_6. They were given 100 milligrams of B_6 daily for three to ten months. It was noted that B_6 helped reduce the frequency and intensity of asthmatic attacks. The belief here is that some attacks of asthma may be traced to an "error" in the metabolism of vitamin B_6. With a supplement, this "error" may be corrected, and resulting in hope for fewer asthma attacks.[24]

Vitamin C Soothes Bronchial Spasms. Researchers were able to ease bronchial spasms in asthmatics by having them take 500 milligrams of vitamin C 90 minutes before exercise. Vitamin C is able to reduce sensitivity to offensive agents in the air, and it also protects some asthmatics against throat spasms.[25]

Still another report has found that taking 1,000 milligrams of vitamin C daily is helpful in reducing sensitivity to noxious irritants in the environment.[26]

Magnesium Is Comforting. Your asthma could be traced to a deficiency of magnesium, a mineral used to comfort asthmatics. In one situation, doctors gave magnesium sulfate intravenously to treat suffering asthmatics and soothe their attacks. It reportedly provided speedy relief. The reason in this instance is that magnesium provides muscle relaxation. Asthma is a violent muscle spasm in the area of the throat and chest. A magnesium supplement of 400 milligrams daily may help boost your resistance to attacks . . . or, at least minimize the reactions.[27]

ATHEROSCLEROSIS

Symptoms

Atherosclerosis is a condition in which the inner layer of the artery wall is made thick and irregular by deposits of fatty substances. These deposits (called atheromata or plaques) project above the surface of the inner layer of the artery, and decrease the diameter of the internal channel of the vessel. This condition is a form of arteriosclerosis, which is characterized by thickening and loss of elasticity of artery walls; this is traced to the accumulation of fibrous tissue, fatty substances (lipids). The problem is that the small blood cells do not know when to stop clumping. They build a blockage from blood cells, cholesterol, and fatty materials throughout your arterial network, until an atheroma (patch) bulges out from the arterial wall. The dangerous atheroma chokes off your blood flow. Should the artery be further narrowed by stress and smoking (both of which tighten blood vessels), or a buildup of cholesterol, the risk is that congestion will occur. Blood cannot transport oxygen. Once blood is cut off to the brain, there is a high risk for a stroke. If blood is denied to your heart, you could develop angina or a heart attack. Very early warning symptoms include dizzy spells that last for a while and weakness in an arm or leg.

Natural Remedies

To build immunity to atherosclerosis or reverse this life-threatening condition, your initial step should be to reduce your intake of fat. You will help reduce body weight, triglycerides (another type of blood fat), and cholesterol . . . all of which will help keep you free of atherosclerosis.

Basically, fats are divided into two categories:

1. *saturated fats* are found in foods of animal origin. These include the fats in whole milk, cream, cheese, butter, meat, and poultry. Coconut and palm oils are derived from vegetables and are called "tropical oils," but are highly saturated.

2. *unsaturated fats* are found in foods of plant origin. These include vegetable oils such as those from the sunflower, corn, soybean, safflower and other such plants. Some fish are also sources of unsaturated fats.

CAREFUL: Each gram of fat supplies about nine calories, whether saturated or unsaturated. This comes to about 100 calories per tablespoon. So you are not cutting calories by eating margarine instead of butter. However, you will be decreasing your consumption of saturated fat if you make that switch.

Limiting intake of fat will help protect your arteries from the accumulation of atheromata or plaques. Fat is the villain that causes atherosclerosis. Nip the enemy in the bud with your first natural *remedy*: you will reduce the calories you get from fat to about 30 percent of your total caloric intake. *Benefit*: This is a level that is low enough to prevent the buildup of fatty deposits inside your artery walls.

How Much Fat Is in the Food You Eat? Here is a handy "fat-finding formula" that answers your question in a minute. There are nine calories in one gram of fat. To calculate the percentage of fat calories in any food, read the label for grams of fat and calories per serving, then plug into this formula:

$$\frac{\text{Grams of Fat} \times 9}{\text{Total Calories}} \times 100 = \text{percentage of fat calories}$$

Example: A bag of potato chips says each 160-calorie serving has 10 grams of fat. Just multiply those 10 grams by 9 and you have 90. Then divide by total calories (160) and you have 0.56. Multiply by 100, to give the percentage of calories from fat, which equal about 56 percent. *Careful*: You now see that the 10 grams of fat in one "small" ounce of potato chips can be very high, indeed!

To make it easier to count fat grams for your daily ration, base the amount on the amount of calories you take in daily:

Calorie Intake	Grams of Fat
1200*	33
1400*	39
1600*	44
1800	50
2000	56
2200	61
2400	67
2600	72
2800	78

* At these levels, you may fall short of the RDA for essential nutrients and should consider taking a multiple vitamin-and-mineral supplement.

Easy Ways to Reduce Dietary Fat

- Use less fat-containing spreads on breads.
- Eat only three to six ounces of meat a day.
- Be sure to read food labels; select low-fat products.
- Bake, broil or boil foods instead of frying them.
- Broil meats on a rack so excess fat drips into the pan.
- Use non-stick pans to limit the amount of fat needed for cooking.
- Steam vegetables and flavor with herbs and spices instead of butter or margarine.
- Be careful of salad dressings, which may be high in fat. Try making your own using less oil than usual and a bit more vinegar and/or water. Or else, use lemon juice or wine vinegar with little or no oil instead of regular dressing.
- Make recipe changes. Use three-quarters the amount of fat called for. Then reduce the amount to one-half. Many recipes, especially those containing meat, call for more fat than is necessary.
- Avoid high-fat snacks, such as potato chips, cheese, chocolate, ice cream, nuts and seeds. Snack on fresh fruits, vegetable chunks and whole grain crackers made without fat.
- If eating outside, avoid foods that are dipped in batter and deep fried.
- Save 8 grams of fat per cup by drinking skim milk instead of whole.
- Eat baked chicken without the skin rather than fried chicken to save 8 grams of fat per 3-ounce serving.

- When you're at the salad bar ladling on the dressing, remember that each tablespoon has 9 grams of fat.
- Try a cup of frozen yogurt instead of gourmet ice cream to save 20 grams of fat.
- Ten potato chips have 7 grams of fat. Go easy!

Fight Fat with Fish Oils. Keep your fat levels down, and satisfy your taste buds at the same time with more fish. Omega-3 fatty acids found in fish oil will help the fat swim out of your body. Many studies have used about 15 grams of fish oil a day; you can achieve the same fat-washing benefits by eating fish regularly, or by combining a high-fish diet with infrequent use of capsules. *Example:* An 8-ounce serving of mackerel, herring or salmon will give you about the same benefits as about 15 capsules.

Keep your arteries clean with a low-fat program . . . for longer life!

FAT CONTENT OF COMMON FOODS

Food	Portion	Fat (in grams)	Food	Portion	Fat (in grams)
Meat, Fish, Poultry			(cod, flounder, grouper, haddock, pollack, snapper)	3 ounces	1
(cooked weight)					
Beef, trimmed of fat					
Top round	3 ounces	5			
Chuck, pot roast	3 ounces	8	Darker-fleshed (higher fat) (mackerel, salmon, fresh tuna)	3 ounces	5
Porterhouse steak	3 ounces	9			
Reg. ground beef (27% fat*)	3 ounces	18	Tuna, canned in water	3 ounces	1
Lean/ground chuck (20% fat*)	3 ounces	15	Crabmeat	3 ounces	2
			Crab, imitation	3 ounces	1
Extra Lean/ ground round (15% fat*)	3 ounces	12	Shrimp/ Scallops	3 ounces	1
Egg	1	6	Poultry		
Fish			Chicken, light meat, no skin	3 ounces	4
White-fleshed (lowest fat)					

Food	Portion	Fat (in grams)	Food	Portion	Fat (in grams)
Chicken, light meat, with skin	3 ounces	9	Skim	8 ounces	0
			Buttermilk	8 ounces	2
			Chocolate (2% fat)	8 ounces	5
Chicken, dark meat, no skin	3 ounces	8	Evaporated, whole	4 ounces	10
Chicken wing, with skin	3 wings	21	Evaporated, skim	4 ounces	0
Turkey, light meat, no skin	3 ounces	3	Condensed, sweetened	4 ounces	14
			Sherbert	½ cup	2
Pork			Yogurt		
Bacon	6 slices (2 ounces)	28	Lowfat, with fruit	8 ounces	3
Canadian bacon	2 ounces	5	Nonfat, plain	8 ounces	0
Ham, regular (11% fat)	3 ounces	8	Whole milk, plain	8 ounces	7
Pork chop, loin, trimmed	3 ounces	12	Frozen	½ cup	0–3
Sausage, link	1 (2½ ounces)	22	**Fats**		
Veal cutlet	3 ounces	4	Butter	1 teaspoon	4
Luncheon meats			Dip	2 Tbsp.	4–5
Bologna	2 ounces	11	Margarine (stick or soft)	1 teaspoon	4
Hot dog, beef	1 (2 ounces)	16	Margarine-like spread (60% fat)	1 teaspoon	3
Liverwurst	2 ounces	16	Mayonnaise, regular	1 teaspoon	4
Dairy Products			Mayonnaise, reduced fat (light)	1 teaspoon	2
Cheese			Oil, vegetable	1 teaspoon	5
American	1 ounce	9	Salad dressing		
Cheddar	1 ounce	9	Blue cheese/Oil and vinegar	1 Tbsp.	8
Cottage (4% fat)	½ cup	5	French/1000 Island/ Ranch	1 Tbsp.	6
Cream	1 ounce	10	Italian	1 Tbsp.	7
Mozzarella, part skim	1 ounce	5	Reduced Calorie	1 Tbsp.	1–4
Swiss	1 ounce	8	Shortening, vegetable	1 teaspoon	4
Cream, heavy	½ cup	44			
Ice cream, rich	½ cup	15	**Baked Goods**		
Ice cream, regular (10% fat)	½ cup	7	Biscuit, baking powder	1	5
Ice milk	½ cup	3			
Milk					
Whole	8 ounces	8			
Lowfat, 2%	8 ounces	5			

Food	Portion	Fat (in grams)	Food	Portion	Fat (in grams)
Bread: white, wheat, rye	1 slice	1	Olives	4 medium	4
Cake			Vegetables, most kinds, plain	¾ cup	0
Angel food	1 piece	0	Broccoli, plain	¾ cup	0
Boston cream pie	3½ ounces	10	Broccoli, w/ 2 Tbsp. cheese or hollandaise sauce	¾	5–9
Cheesecake	3½ ounces	11–16			
Chocolate with chocolate icing	3½ ounces	18	Potato, baked, plain	1 med (3½ ounces)	0
Spongecake, no icing	3½ ounces	6	Potato, french-fried	20 (3½ ounces)	9–17
Cookies			Dried beans (kidney, garbanzo, etc.)	½ cup cooked	1
Animal crackers	7	1			
Brownie with nuts	2" × 2"	6–10			
Chocolate chip	2 medium	6	**Nuts and Seeds**		
Chocolate sandwich	2	4	Cashews (1¼ ounces)	4 Tbsp.	16
Gingersnap	6 small	2	Peanuts (1¼ ounces)	4 Tbsp.	18
Oatmeal raisin	2 medium	5	Peanut butter	1 Tbsp.	8
Vanilla wafers	6	4	Sunflower seeds (1¼ ounces)	4 Tbsp.	19
Crackers, graham	2 squares	2			
Crackers, saltines	4	1			
Crackers, rye wafers	2 long	0–1	**Snacks and Miscellaneous**		
Doughnut	1	6–9			
Muffin, from mix	1 small	4	Chocolate bar, plain	1 ounce	9
Pie, cream/custard type	⅛ of 9" pie	12–18	Pâté de foie gras	4 ounces	50
Pie, fruit type	⅛ of 9" pie	9–17	Popcorn (popped in oil)	1 cup	1
Cereals, Grains, Pasta			Potato chips	1 ounce (14)	11
Cereal, most ready-to-eat	1 cup	1	Pretzels	1 ounce (6)	1
Macaroni	½ cup	0	Soup, canned beef noodle	1 cup	3
Macaroni and cheese	½ cup	9	Soup, canned cream of mushroom, w/ water	1 cup	9
Noodles, egg	½ cup	1			
Oatmeal, cooked	½ cup	1	Sugar/Honey/Jelly	1 Tbsp.	0
Rice	½ cup	0			
Fruits and Vegetables					
Fruit juice	½ cup	0			
Fresh fruit, most kinds	1 piece	0			
Avocado	½	15			

* Average value. Percent of fat will vary somewhat between states.

FAT CONTENT OF COMMON FAST FOODS

Food	Fat (in grams)
Arby's	
Regular roast beef	15
Junior roast beef	9
Beef 'n Cheddar	27
Ham 'n Cheese	14
Turkey Deluxe	17
Superstuffed potato, deluxe	30
Burger King	
Bacon double cheeseburger	31
Chicken salad	4
Hamburger	12
Whopper Sandwich	36
Dairy Queen	
DQ cone, regular	7
DQ dip cone, regular	16
Peanut buster parfait	34
Brazier chili dog	20
Hounder chili dog	41
Fish fillet	18
Chicken breast fillet	34
Onion rings	16
Domino's Pizza	
Cheese pizza, 16" (2 slices)	10
Pepperoni pizza, 16" (2 slices)	18
Deluxe pizza, 16" (2 slices)	20
Hardee's	
Chicken stix (6 pieces)	10
Chicken fillet sandwich	16
Fisherman's fillet	25
Steak biscuit	29
Seafood salad	2
Jack in the Box	
Breakfast Jack sandwich	13
Supreme crescent	40
Hamburger	11

Food	Fat (in grams)
Jumbo Jack Hamburger	34
Chicken fajita pita	8
Taco salad	31
Super Taco	17
Apple turnover	24
Kentucky Fried Chicken	
Original recipe dinner (wing + thigh)	31
(side breast)	16
Extra crispy dinner (wing + thigh)	42
(side breast)	24
Buttermilk biscuit	12
Cole slaw	7
McDonald's	
Egg McMuffin	11
Hotcakes with butter and syrup	9
Hamburger	10
Cheeseburger	14
Quarterpounder with cheese	29
McDLT	37
Filet-O-Fish	27
Chicken McNuggets (6 pieces)	16
McChicken	29
Chicken Oriental Salad (plain)	3
Oriental salad dressing (1 pkt.)	0
French fries, regular	12
Apple pie	14
McDonaldland cookies	11
Vanilla shake	8
Pizza Hut	
Cheese pizza, thin 'n crispy, medium (2 slices)	17
Pepperoni personal pan pizza	29
Taco Bell	
Bean burrito	10
Beef burrito	17
Burrito supreme	19
Taco	11
Chicken fajita	10

Food	Fat (in grams)	Food	Fat (in grams)
Nachos, regular	18	Chicken sandwich	19
Taco salad	62	Stuffed potato, bacon & cheese	30
Seafood salad	41	Chef salad	9
		Taco salad	37
Wendy's		Salad dressings, various reg. (1 Tbsp.)	6–9
		various reduced calorie (1 Tbsp.)	2–4
Single hamburger (¼ pound)	16	Chili	9
Double hamburger	34	Frosty dairy dessert (1 medium)	18
Double cheeseburger	48		
Bacon Swiss burger	44		
Philly Swiss burger	24		

ATHLETE'S FOOT

Symptoms

These vary from one person to another. Itching is the most common symptom and can often signal the start of an infection. Other symptoms include redness, burning, itching, stinging, scaling, and/or peeling. Infected skin can also become inflamed, cracked or blistered. Athlete's foot usually strikes between the toes . . . often between the fourth and fifth toes. It may then spread to the soles and sides of the feet and to toenails. Once toenails become infected, it is difficult to get rid of the infection completely, so prompt and proper treatment is important. Infection is most likely to occur in warm months, when people sweat, and in areas of the skin with small cracks. Athlete's foot (its official name is *tinea pedis*) is caused by a species of *Trichophyton* fungus that invade the skin. To strike, the microscopic fungi need a certain environment. Thus, feet, with 125,000 sweat glands per foot and production of up to a half pint of perspiration a day, become prime breeding grounds. Warm weather and/or continually wearing the same shoes contribute to keeping feet moist and vulnerable.

Why Does It Happen? Common fungal infections are easily transmitted from person to person. Athlete's foot is most commonly contracted by walking barefoot on floors where the fungi are present. Shoes and socks are also likely breeding grounds. Perspiration caused by hot, humid weather, exercise, obesity or tight-fitting clothing and footwear creates the moist environment fungi thrive on. The accumulation of moisture also can soften the skin enough to allow fungi to penetrate it more easily. So although sweaty feet are not the cause of athlete's foot, they may make you more susceptible to picking up a fungal infection.

Older People Susceptible to the Infection. As skin ages, it becomes thinner and drier and, therefore, more susceptible to cracking and other damage that reduces its effectiveness as a barrier to fungal infections. Older people also are more likely to have less efficient immune systems, be predisposed to diabetes, or suffer from pure nutrition—all factors that make them more vulnerable to fungal infections.

Natural Remedies

Six Steps to Ease-Eliminate Athlete's Foot. A set of natural remedies is offered by Dr. Barry H. Block, a practicing doctor of podiatric medicine, in New York City:

1. Choose a shoe made of natural materials such as leather and canvas to allow moisture to escape and let the foot "breathe."

2. Apply a little cornstarch to your shoes before and after wearing them. Cornstarch is more absorbent than talc and contains fewer impurities.

3. Keep your shoes dry. Do not wear them on consecutive days. It takes two to three days for a shoe to adequately dry out. One way you can accelerate this process is to use your hair dryer for a few minutes at a medium heat setting. Another method is to stuff your shoes with old newspapers. Leaving your shoes near a heater is less desirable because it may cause the leather of the shoe to shrink.

4. Clean your feet thoroughly at least twice a day. Fungi are parasites which survive by "eating" the outside layer of your dead skin. Soap and water help to remove this layer. Be sure to thoroughly dry your feet afterward, paying particular attention to the web spaces in between your toes.

5. Change your socks at least twice a day. If your feet tend to sweat, select stockings with a high cotton content. Cotton serves to "wick" moisture to the surface which helps keep your feet cool and dry.

6. If you have a tendency toward fungal infections, apply an over-the-counter talcum powder, as recommended by your podiatrist, daily to your shoes and socks.[28]

Prompt Care Is Vital. Do not neglect athlete's foot. "It can be dangerous!" warns Marvin Sandler, D.P.M., Chief of Podiatry Surgery at Sacred Heart Hospital, in Allentown, Pennsylvania. "When the skin is broken, bacteria enters and causes a secondary infection. An untreated bacterial infection can become very serious if it spreads to other parts of the body through the bloodstream or lymphatic drainage system."[29]

Tips, Remedies, Foot Treatments. Dr. Sandler urges, "The key point is to keep the areas between your toes as dry as possible. Feet should be dried carefully after showering—particularly between the toes. Use of powder can help the feet remain dry. The trick is to rub the powder in; sprinkling it is not effective. Baby powder is good. Finely ground talc is acceptable, if it does not cake. Try to avoid shoes with synthetic uppers. These tend to be nonporous and prevent perspiration from evaporating. It is also preferable to wear shoes with leather soles. *Important:* When drying after a shower, feet should be wiped last! Wiping feet first may infect other parts of the body, particularly the groin (where it can cause 'jock itch')."[29]

Since athlete's foot is contagious, take precautions in public places. Wear thongs in public showers and at poolside. Never wear other peoples' shoes.

One good suggestion is to dry your feet with paper towels that can be thrown away!

Give Your Feet a "Salt Soak." Soak your feet in a mixture of two teaspoons salt per pint of warm water. Enjoy the comforting soak for 10 to 15 minutes at a time. Repeat several times a day. The saline solution rejects the fungus and also eases excessive perspiration.

The Baking Soda Remedy. Add a little lukewarm water to one tablespoon of baking soda and make into a paste. Rub gently on the site of your fungus, especially between your toes. Rinse and dry thoroughly. Dust on some powder.

Air Your Feet. While your shoes are being aired out in the sun for a while, treat your feet to some open air for a few minutes before putting on socks and shoes. **TIP:** Hold a hair dryer about seven inches from your foot, wiggle your toes and let the breeze dry your feet for about 10 minutes. An "air bath" is healthy—for shoes, socks and feet. Your entire body, too!

⋅• B •⋅

BACKACHE

Symptoms

An acute pain strikes suddenly and viciously. You may feel a muscle pull on your back when you try to do ordinary tasks. A chronic pain is one that keeps recurring and hurts for days or weeks. In more serious situations, you could be confined to a chair or bed for an extended period of time. You may have accompanying pain, numbness, tingling or weakness in your extremities. Something has gone wrong with your backbone! Your spine cannot always meet the stress and strain of daily living without something going wrong. You subject your back to a constant pull of gravity upon the vertical and upright spinal column. This places a constant strain on the joints and discs of your vertebrae. Unlike the four-legged creature who carries his spine around in a horizontal position, your spine must support most of your bodyweight when you sit, stand or perform activities. In this vertical position, your lower spinal segment is subjected to more weight bearing than your upper part. You face the stresses of vertebral compression. Unless you are very careful, you could develop disorders or distortions that can hurt . . . and really hurt!

Natural Remedies

To help take the pressure off your hurting back, Dr. Jack Soltanoff, chiropractor, in West Hurley, New York has these natural remedies:

At Home. Lie on a rug or padded floor. Support your neck with a small pillow or rolled up towel. Place another pillow under your knees. Keep hips tilted back and your back against the floor. Hold this position five to ten minutes after the pain goes away.

At Work. Sit with head and back straight. Raise both shoulders to your ears. Hold for 10 seconds. Raise both arms upwards towards the ceiling. Hold 10 seconds. Repeat three times.

Pelvic Tilt. Lie on the floor with knees bent; squeeze buttocks together; pull in abdomen tilting, your pelvis upward. Try to flatten your lower back to the floor. Hold for 10 seconds. Repeat five times.

Partial Sit-up. Lie on your back, knees slightly bent. Criss-cross arms on your chest, slowly lifting head and shoulders off the floor 45 degrees. Count out loud to 10 and slowly lower head and shoulders. Repeat ten times.

Hamstring Stretch. Lie on floor with knees bent. Bring right knee toward your chest, then straighten leg toward ceiling, until your knee is locked. Count out loud to 10 and slowly lower your leg to the floor while keeping your knee straight. Bring your right knee back to starting position. Repeat with your left leg. Alternate your legs. Repeat five times for each leg.

Knee to Chest Lift. Lie on the floor, both knees bent. Grasp right leg below your knee and pull towards your right shoulder. Hold for 10 seconds. Repeat five times. Alternate legs.

Safe Lifting to Protect Your Back

Dr. Soltanoff tells us, "You can ease pressure on your spinal column and avoid a backache if you follow the basics of safer lifting. Here is a five-step plan I give to my patients, and the results are wonderful."

1. Get a firm footing, with your feet apart for a good balance. Stand close to the load. Squat (don't bend waist). Take a deep breath. Tighten your stomach muscles to help support your back under the load.
2. Life with your legs—they're much stronger than your back. Bring your back to the vertical position.
3. Hold the load close to your body; this puts less pressure on your back.
4. If you have to turn, do so with your feet and **not** by twisting your back.
5. Put the load down again by squatting, **not** by bending your back. Keep your fingers out from under the load.

"If you have to lift from a height above your shoulders, limit yourself to a light load. Otherwise, stand on a sturdy, steady platform to bring your shoulders above the load. **Always** test weight by pushing up against the load before picking it up. And ask for help, rather than risk an injured back," advises Dr. Soltanoff.[30]

How to "Ice" Away Your Back Pain. If you experience a painful flare-up, try an ice remedy. An ice pack on the location of the pain for about 10 minutes will help shrink swelling and ease the strain that is hurting your back muscles. TIP: Quicker relief is enjoyed if you massage the hurt area with the ice pack!

Healing Heat Soothes Bad Back. After three days of the ice remedy, change to heat for fulfillment of pain relief. Put a soft towel in a bowl of very warm water. Wring it thoroughly. Flatten it so no creases are seen. Lie face down; put pillows beneath your hips and ankles so you are raised slightly. Fold the warm towel across the painful section of your back. Cover with some plastic wrap. Put a heating pad (medium level) on top of the plastic. Then put a comfortable weight on top of all this—such as a heavy book. The point is to create gentle but firm pressure. The medium heat will spread warmth through your back, coupled with some moisture that soothes and comforts muscle spasms. Only 30 minutes and this natural remedy should help do away with the hurt of your back.

First Ice, Then Heat . . . Double Benefits. A contrast will be extremely beneficial. Try 30 minutes of ice, then switch to 30 minutes of heat. Keep repeating this contrast. It helps soothe the most stubborn of backaches.

Poor Sleeping Posture May Cause Bad Back. You harm your back without realizing it by sleeping incorrectly. Come morning and you find it difficult or impossible to roll out of bed. To remedy this problem, sleep with your body in good alignment. Let pillows help support your body.

If You Sleep on Your Side. Choose a firm, fairly thick pillow for your head and neck to prevent your head from dropping down toward the mattress. For a low-back problem, place a second pillow between your knees to prevent pull on your lower back. TIP: If your problem area is in your neck or shoulders, place a small pillow in front of you to support the arm that is uppermost, so it does not drop forward and pull on your neck and upper back.

If You Sleep on Your Back. Place a comfortable pillow under your head and one or two large pillows under your knees.

If You Must Sleep on Your Stomach. This is not a desirable position, but if unavoidable, place a pillow under your stomach to protect your back from arching. Or else, bend one leg up to the side so that you are slightly raised on that side, and place a pillow partially under your stomach and chest to support the part of you that is raised. **CAREFUL:** In either position for sleeping on your stomach, do **not** use a pillow under your head since this tilts your head backwards and will compress your neck.

Lumber Is Good to Your Lower Back. Your bed may have a slight sag in the middle that could give you a low-back pain in the morning. A piece of plywood inserted between the mattress and the boxspring helps firm up foundation and protect you against low back pain. You'll sleep better, too!

Hints, Tips, Remedies. Take frequent stand-up breaks throughout the day if you find yourself sitting too long. When you sit, guard against slumping by inserting a three-inch small pillow behind your back. To avoid slouching when you sit, perch at the base of your buttocks with a support at your lower back. Lighten up on bundles you carry; divide the weight equally between both arms. If you use a shoulder bag, switch sides frequently. If you use a typewriter or computer, make sure the machine or screen is at eye-level. Use a book stand to copy from instead of letting the material lie flat on your desk.

CASE HISTORY—*Soothes Hurtful Back with Tender Loving Remedies*

Recurring back pain that made Janet R. cry out with sobbing hurt when she got up in the morning, just refused to go away. She had responsibilities at home and also at a part-time job that offered opportunities, but the shooting spasms made her bedridden so often, she feared incapacitation and loss of a pending promotion. Medications did ease the symptoms but she did not want to become addicted to pain killers. She wanted to end the dilemma. She sought advice from a visiting chiropractor, who delivered an important lecture on how to be good to your bad back. She managed to make it to the lecture hall; afterwards, Janet R. made an appointment. The chiropractor told her how to improve her posture, then pointed to poor sleeping posture as a basic cause of her painful back. She used the pillows as described previously; she also used the ice and heat remedies to ease the spasms. Within nine days, her back was flexible. The pain was gone! She could resume obligations with energy and enthusiasm . . . and was given the coveted promotion on her job. She was free of the hurt, thanks to the tender loving remedies. Natural, too!

BREATHING DIFFICULTIES

Symptoms

Unable to get a deep breath, shortness of breath, shallow breathing, rapid inhalation, trouble getting enough air, as well as breathlessness, are different ways of describing this symptom. If you have trouble exhaling, it could mean asthma. If there is trouble getting air in, as well as recurring gasps or sighs, it may be anxiety. More serious conditions related to breathing difficulties include bronchitis, emphysema or chronic obstructive lung disease (COLD). Poor breathing may be a symptom of heart problems. If your master pump, your heart, is not pumping efficiently, blood starts accumulating in the millions of tiny lung capillaries, swelling them stiff with retained fluid. This fluid interferes with close contact between air and blood. Oxygen you have just inhaled cannot get to your bloodstream. You gasp for air!

Natural Remedies

To boost your circulation, speedy relief for better breathing includes:

Pillow Prop. While in bed, prop yourself up with pillows to make it easier for you to inhale-exhale healthfully.

Leg Movement. Whether you sit or lie, keep your legs moving as much as is convenient. You will boost your sluggish circulation and send more oxygen throughout your system.

Daily Walk. At least 60 minutes a day or about one (or more) mile walk. This helps accelerate your body's ability to use oxygen.

Avoid Salt. A salt-free diet helps take the pressure off your heart by reducing the amount of fluid it has to pump. Less salt means better breathing . . . and a healthier heart, too.

Circulation-Boosting Breathing Exercise. Dr. Jack Soltanoff, chiropractor of West Hurley, New York, offers an easy exercise that "influences your breathing and circulatory centers. I have been able to correct breathing difficulties in many of my patients with this oxygen-booster." He explains:

Inhale slowly through your nose; at the same time, slightly stick out your lower abdomen which you then slightly take in—your ribs should be lifted outwards and upwards toward your chest. Fill your lungs *completely* with air, but without strain. Hold your breath for two seconds only.

Then (and this is important) exhale through your mouth *on the sustained note of OO.* Your lips must form the roundest possible O and the air must be exhaled slowly to the utmost limit, but again *without strain.*

Repeat this remedy for 10 minutes, three times a day at first. Work up to no more than 15 minutes a day, when the remedy is done four times daily. *NOTE:* You may do this Circulation-Boosting Breathing Exercise while standing or sitting.

Suggestion: Dr. Soltanoff suggests, "This exercise should be carried out every day, preferably immediately after a meal, since it will help in digestion and regularity. The key here is persistence; regular application. To relieve the possible monotony of the sustained OO-ing sound, the OO-ing can take the form of a scale or tune."[31]

Hyperventilation Can Be Controlled. Overbreathing or "breathing fast" is usually traced to stress or anxiety. Hyperventilation may be a symptom of pneumonia, a blood infection or a heart problem. Mostly, anxiety is the cause. You breathe rapidly and deeply, although you do not require the additional oxygen. You exhale much carbon dioxide, which causes the blood to become alkaline; a panic attack may follow. A typical episode of hyperventilation is about 30 minutes. To help control:

Paper Bag Remedy. Rebreathing into a paper bag will replace the lost carbon dioxide and restore balance. It also gives a sense of comfort.

Calm Down. To slow your breathing, sit down and relax. Balance your breathing rate. One breath every six seconds . . . or ten breaths per minute. This simple remedy helps stabilize your breathing.

Exercise, Caffeine, Smoking. Regular exercise helps decrease anxiety so that you breathe much better. Avoid caffeine, which is a stimulating trigger for hyperventilation. The same reaction occurs with smoking because nicotine is an artificial stimulant that upsets your breathing rates. Omit caffeine and smoking, and you should have healthier breathing.

Nutritional Remedies for Breathing Difficulties

Robert H. Garrison, Jr., R.Ph., and Elizabeth Somer, M.A., R.D., co-authors of *The Nutrition Desk Reference* point out, "Good Nutrition helps maintain healthy lung tissue by strengthening the immune system and increasing the body's resistance to infection and disease, maintaining a healthy epithelial lining, and deactiviting free radicals and other highly reactive compounds that might damage lung tissue and possibly cause cancer."

Vitamin A and Beta-Carotene. The researchers point out, "Vitamin A and its precursor beta-carotene are essential for the normal development and maintenance of epithelial tissue and mucous membranes, including the lining of the lungs, bronchi and other respiratory tissues. These epithelial tissues form a barrier to bacteria and other pathogens and aid in the prevention of infection and disease. Vitamin A and beta-carotene also contribute to a well-functioning influence on resistance to lung disorders."[32]

Vitamin E. The antioxidant effects help protect cell membranes in the lungs from damage caused by air pollutants and tobacco smoke. Vitamin E is found in nuts and seeds, wheat germ and cold-pressed vegetable oil.

Vitamin B Complex. Adequate amounts of Vitamin B_1, Vitamin B_2, Vitamin B_6, folic acid and Vitamin B_{12} are also needed for immune boosting and lung strengthening, say medical researchers. In addition, pantothenic acid is needed to build resistance to respiratory tract infection.[33]

Minerals. Iron, manganese, zinc and copper are several minerals needed for the maintenance of a strong immune system and protection of all tissues, especially in the lungs, to form a barrier to the polluted environment.

Foods for Breathing Difficulties. Boost intake of carrots, dark green leafy vegetables, apricots, other dark green or orange fruits and vegetables. Include cooked dried beans and peas, low-fat or non-fat dairy products, such as milk and yogurt.

You can live for weeks without food, days without water, but you cannot survive more than a few minutes without air. All 60 trillion cells in your body need oxygen. Your breathing system needs to be kept in good working order . . . to keep you alive and healthy! With better care and nutrition, you can breathe new life into your body and mind!

BRONCHITIS

Symptoms

Inflammation of the bronchi (air passage beyond the trachea or windpipe that has cartilage and mucus glands in the wall). Acute bronchitis is caused by viruses or bacteria and is characterized by coughing, production of sputum, and narrowing of the bronchi because of spasmodic contraction. Chronic bronchitis is noted by coughing up excessive mucus and difficulty in catching breath.

Natural Remedies

Be good to your lungs. Avoid irritants such as tobacco smoke, perfume, air pollution and fumes from common household cleaners and paint. *Note:* If you are strong enough to cough, use steam or mist from a vaporizer to help make your breathing easier.

Avoid Smoking. This cannot be emphasized enough. Nine out of 10 cases of bronchitis are traced to smoking. Not only should you quit this habit, you should also quit being near others who smoke. "Passive smoking" is about as dangerous as if you inhaled a cigarette in your mouth!

More Liquids Will Ease Symptoms. Six glasses of liquids daily will make your mucus more watery and easier to expel. Avoid temperature extremes, which tend to irritate your bronchial tubes and related lung tissues. Comfortably warm and comfortably cool liquids are helpful. Plain water is soothing. Avoid alcoholic or caffeine beverages because they are diuretics and cause more fluid loss . . . when you need to have more fluid for your lungs.

Steam Away Coughing Spells. Fill your bathroom sink with hot water. Make a towel tent over your head and the sink, and inhale the steam for ten minutes every five hours.

Milk: Does It Cause Problems? Dairy products may thicken mucus and cause distress in some situations. If you find this to be true in your case, cut down on intake of milk and other dairy foods and see if that will resolve the problem. Take a 1,000 milligram calcium supplement daily to replace that which is found in dairy foods. For better absorption, take closer to bedtime.

Vitamin C Builds Strong Immunity. About 1,000 milligrams of vitamin C daily will help build immunity to offensive pollutants in the air and control the incidence of bronchial spasm. This vitamin strengthens the breathing apparatus so that there is less reaction to noxious agents and easing of throat spasms. Vitamin C is also found in citrus fruits, juices, broccoli, Brussels sprouts, green peppers, kale, turnip greens, guava, and strawberries. In food preparation or processing, the vitamin C content of food can be lowered, hence the suggestion for a daily supplement.

CASE HISTORY—*Simple Changes Bring Bronchitis to a Halt*

George A. felt that recurring bronchitis attacks were cutting into his responsibilities as a truck fleet dispatcher. He had been "grounded" to a desk job because he frequently broke out into choking, hacking coughs that forced him to pull over to the curb to avoid an accident. The bronchial attacks made it impossible to drive safely, if at all. He was considered a risk on the road. In the office, he had to take frequent breaks because of coughing attacks that left him exhausted. He had to catch his breath upon the slightest exertion on the job or at home. Medications offered some relief, but he was still vulnerable to hacking coughs that left him gasping for precious air.

A visiting salesman told him of some natural remedies that would help restore resistance to the bronchitis. George A. had tried everything, but he decided to try these remedies. He shunned everyone who smoked, even wore a button that said, "Smoke? Keep back!" Then he took at least six to eight glasses of plain water daily, among other liquids. He quit all alcohol and caffeine beverages, which he previously liked. Then he reduced his milk intake. He would use the steam treatment at home every night. (It helped him sleep and awaken better.) In the morning, another steam treatment. With 1,000 milligrams daily of vitamin C, George A. experienced relief within two weeks and had fewer bronchial attacks. By the end of eight weeks, his attacks were few and far between. Still, he felt reluctant to go back on the road; he held a part-time truck route without suffering any coughing breakdown. Soon, he could look ahead to returning to full-time road work. The natural remedies helped bring bronchitis to a halt!

BRUISES

Symptoms

A bruise or contusion is an area of skin discoloration caused by the escape of blood from ruptured underlying vessels following injury. Initially red or pink, a bruise gradually becomes bluish, then greenish-yellow, as the hemoglobin in the tissues breaks down chemically and is absorbed. If the bruises are of a tiny, pinhead size, they are called *purpura*. If the bruises are larger and more extensive, they are called *ecchymosis*. The elderly often have *senile purpura*. Be alert to any discoloration of or swelling beneath the skin. If bruises appear all over the body, they are symptoms of other illnesses that call for medical attention.

Natural Remedies

The sooner you treat a bruise, the quicker the healing. Fast remedies include:

Ice Away the Hurtful Bruise. Apply ice as quickly as possible after the injury. The application should remain to prevent a bruise. Ice constricts the capillaries and slows the bleeding and swelling. Less blood spills into the tissues to cause a big blotch. *How to use ice*: Apply an ice pack at 15-minute intervals. Do not apply heat in between but let your skin warm naturally. Do this for about 24 hours. An old-fashioned ice bag is soothing. Or else, wrap a small container of frozen food in a towel and apply to the injured arm. You'll need a few such containers if they defrost too rapidly.

Use Heat After 24 Hours of Ice. A comfortably hot bag is soothing on the hurt area after your 24-hour ice treatment. *Benefit*: the heat opens blood vessels and boosts circulation in the region.

Raise the Injured Foot. You have hurt your foot . . . or leg . . . or thigh. You want quick relief and less risk of a bruise. Lift up your injured limb. Better yet, do more standing . . . or walking, without hurting the area. **Benefit**: Bruises are small pockets of blood. Like any liquid, blood runs downhill. You need to prevent the blood from accumulating in a bruise. When you lift your foot (or stand in comfort or take a walk), the gathered blood makes its way down through your soft tissues to different parts of your body. The injury is healed all the better . . . faster, naturally, too.

Vitamin C Builds Resistance to Bruises. If you are deficient in this vitamin, you tend to bruise more easily. Your wounds take longer to heal. Vitamin C raises plasma and leukocyte (white blood cells that promote healing) levels, reducing incidence of bruising, while improving the immune system, too. Vitamin C helps build protective collagen tissue around the blood vessels of your skin. About 1,000 milligrams of vitamin C daily will help to protect you against bruises and promote better healing, if you should bruise.

Zap Bruises with Zinc. Elderly people are often found to be deficient in zinc, needed to enhance the immune system. Zinc helps protect against the "purple spot" bruising (purpura) that seems indigenous among older adults. Adequate zinc on a daily basis is needed to attack bruises . . . before they occur and also after they occur. Zinc is found in wheat germ, wheat bran, cooked cowpeas (blackeye). The RDA is a minimum of 15 milligrams for adults. Zinc is also available as a supplement.

Bioflavonoids. Found in the membrane lining of citrus fruits, this is a group of nutrients that help heal bruises, blemishes and skin disorders. If you have severe bruises that keep occuring, your skin will benefit from 5,000 milligrams of bioflavonoids daily. They will help restore the strength of the support structure of your skin and also accelerate the healing process.

Check Your Medications. If you take aspirin to protect against heart trouble, you'll find a bump becomes a bruise very easily. Other medications such as blood thinners, anti-inflammatory products, anti-depressants, asthma medicines can inhibit clotting beneath the skin and lead to larger bruises.

——————————————————— ❧ ———————————————————

CASE HISTORY—*"Age Bruises" Respond to Nutritional Healers*

Ordinary housework with its usual bumps against furniture gave Ruth O'C. a bad case of bruises. If she hit her arm against a doorway, she broke out in so-called age bruises that were reddish-bluish in color. At age 76, she wondered if bruises were part of getting old. Not so, said her dermatologist who prescribed a food program with increased fresh fruits and vegetables and more whole grains. He also told Ruth O'C. to take 1,000 milligrams of vitamin C daily. She boosted her immune system until she was no longer so fragile and her age bruises were resisted. Nutritional healers had boosted her skin structure to protect against bruises.

BURNS

Symptoms

Burns come in several classifications:

First-degree burns injure the outside layer of the skin. Brief contact with hot objects, hot water or steam are common symptoms that cause no blistering of the area. There may be redness, mild swelling, pain.

Second-degree burns injure layers of the skin beneath its surface. Brief contact with hot liquids, flash burns from gasoline and other substances cause the burns. There may be redness, or blotchy or streaky appearance, blisters, and swelling that will last for several days; also moist, oozy appearance of the skin surface, with pain.

Third-degree burns will destroy all layers of the skin. Common causes are fire, prolonged contact with hot substances and electrical burns. The burned area appears white or destroyed. There is destroyed skin. Little pain is felt because nerve endings have been destroyed.

Natural Remedies

Your first goal is to *put out the fire! FAST!!!* Immediately—

Extinguish the Fire. For minor burns, flush the affected parts with lots and lots of cold water. At least 20 minutes or until the burning stops. Do NOT use ice or ice water, which worsens the burn. For a contact burn, run the hurt part under cold water. If you have been splattered by hot grease or hot soup, remove the soiled clothing first. Then wash the grease off your skin. Soak the burn in cold water. **CARE-FUL:** If the clothing sticks to the skin, rinse water over the clothing, and go to a medical facility. Do NOT pull the clothing off or you will cause more damage.

DANGER: Butter Is Harmful. Never use butter or any other food on a burn since such items will seal heat in your tissue and compound the problem, possibly cause infection. NO vinegar, honey, or vegetable peelings, either.

Simple Burn Covering. After the burn is washed, cover with a clean, dry cloth; a thick gauze pad is comforting. A dry, sterile dressing is helpful. Do not touch the area for 24 hours.

Washing Your Burn. After 24 hours, wash the burned area gently with mild soap and water once a day. Keep the area dry, covered and clean between washings . . . and do not touch it.

Aloe Cools, Heals. Aloe vera plant is soothing and healing to your burn. An over-the-counter aloe cream or lotion (available at health stores) will provide an analgesic or pain-relieving reaction to comfort and cool your burn. (Best not to use aloe if you are taking blood thinners or have been diagnosed with cardiovascular problems.)

Vitamin E Soothes, Restores Health. After several days, when your burn is healing, soothe and boost the process with vitamin E. Break open a capsule and rub the liquid onto the affected area. Feels good and helps protect against scarring.

Hands Off Any Blisters. Those pop-up bubbles form a bandage made by Nature. Don't touch them. If a blister opens on its own, clean the area with soap and water, gently dab on a little aloe vera lotion and cover.

For More Serious Burns. Put the burned area in cold (not iced) water or apply cold-water compresses (a clean towel, washcloth or hand-kerchief soaked in cold water) until pain subsides. Gently pat the area dry with a clean towel or other soft material. Cover the burned area with a dry, nonfluffy sterile bandage or clean cloth to prevent infection. Seek medical help if very serious. This is important for burns that cover more than 15 percent of the body of an adult or 10 percent of the body of a child, or for burns of the face, hands or feet. To determine the percentage of the burned area, an easy rule is that your hand (including fingers) represents one percent of your body area.

❧ C ❧

CANCER

Symptoms

Cancer is a large group of diseases characterized by uncontrolled growth and spread of abnormal cells. Cancer strikes at any age, more frequently with advancing age. The danger is that cancer invades and destroys normal tissues. The spread may be regional—confined to one region of the body—when cells are trapped by lymph nodes. Cancer may also spread throughout the body and threaten life. The American Cancer Society lists seven warning signals:

1. Change in bowel or bladder habits.
2. A sore that does not heal.
3. Unusual bleeding or discharge.
4. Thickening or lump in breast or elsewhere.
5. Indigestion or difficulty in swallowing.
6. Obvious change in wart or mole.
7. Nagging cough or hoarseness.

Important: If you have one or more warning signals, see your medical specialist.[34]

Natural Remedies

The National Cancer Institute explains, "About 80 percent of cancer cases appear to be linked to the way people live their lives. For example, whether or not you smoke, the foods you eat, and certain industrial pollutants all affect your likelihood of getting cancer. The role of diet in the cause and prevention of cancer is particularly important. About 35 percent of cancer deaths may be associated with dietary influences." The Institute suggests that you might reduce your cancer risk by following these recommendations:

1. **Avoid** *Obesity*. If you are 40 percent or more overweight, you increase your risk of colon, breast, prostate, gallbladder, ovary, and uterine cancer.

2. *Cut Down on Total Fat Intake.* High fat intake may be a factor in the development of certain cancers, particularly breast, colon and prostate. By avoiding fatty foods, you are better able to control body weight.

3. *Eat More High-Fiber Foods.* These include whole grain breads and cereals, fruits and vegetables and legumes such as dry peas and beans. These foods may help to reduce the risk of colon cancer. Furthermore, high fiber foods are a wholesome substitution for fatty foods.

4. *Include Foods Rich in Vitamins A and C.* Favorable foods are dark green and deep yellow fresh vegetables and fruits, such as carrots, yams, peaches and apricots for beta-carotene, the predecessor of vitamin A. Also use oranges, grapefruits, strawberries, and green and red peppers for vitamin C. These foods may help lower risk for cancers of the larynx, esophagus, and the lungs.

5. *Daily Intake of Cruciferous Vegetables.* These are cabbage, broccoli, Brussels sprouts, kohlrabi and cauliflower, among others. They have ingredients that build resistance to certain cancers. Cruciferous vegetables are identified by their flowers with four leaves in the pattern of a cross.

6. *Avoid Salt-cured, Smoked or Nitrite-cured Foods.* Among those who eat these foods frequently, there is more incidence of cancer of the esophagus and stomach. Best to avoid such foods.

7. *Keep Alcohol Consumption Moderate if You Must Drink.* Heavy use of alcohol, especially when accompanied by cigarette smoking or smokeless tobacco, increases risk of cancers of the mouth, larynx, throat, esophagus, and liver. Alcoholic drinks are high in calories and very low in vitamins and minerals. It is best to avoid alcohol . . . and smoking. You will then strengthen your immune system to resist many types of cancer.[35]

Immune Boosting Remedies. You can diminish cancer risks through immune boosting remedies. Maintain proper weight. Limit your intake of fat. More carbohydrates as substitutes for high-fat foods will control weight. Choose lean cuts of meat; trim away all visible fat prior to cooking.

"Poultry offers another healthy low-fat choice, provided you take simple precautions," says Tricia Smith, R.N., Coordinator for the Cancer Prevention Clinic of the University of Wisconsin Cancer Center, in Madison. "When preparing poultry, cut away skin and other visible fat before cooking. If you grill, keep the flame low and cook the meat longer since studies show charred meat as well as smoke and grease may contain compounds thought to cause cancer.

"Changing your cooking methods can also help reduce fat intake. Roasting, boiling, steaming or microwaving are preferable to pan or deep-fat frying. If you do fry, use non-stick cooking sprays, low in saturated fats. Better yet, plan meals around low-fat dairy products, fresh fruits and vegetables and whole grain products high in fiber."

Is Fiber Essential? "Definitely, says Tricia Smith, R.N. "Fiber helps speed food through your digestive system, to protect your body from colon and rectal cancer. Fruits and vegetables, common fiber sources, also contain vitamins A, C, and E, and minerals that inhibit cancer from developing."

Tips On Salads. Smith suggests, "Salads make a healthy meal but be careful against heaping on high-fat dressings. Use low calorie dressings, or better yet, oil and vinegar or lemon juice. If you nsist on richer dressings, put just a little on the side."

Nutrition Is Cancer Fighter. "Include more fruits and vegetables in your diet," urges Roswell Boutwell, M.D., Professor of Oncology, University of Wisconsin Medical School. "For example, studies show garlic, onions, cabbage and Brussels sprouts help protect laboratory animals from various types of cancer. Plus, vitamins in green and yellow vegetables are great inhibitors of carcinogens. They prevent certain biochemical changes in the body that can increase the risks of getting cancer. There's enough evidence to indicate that a well-balanced diet—which includes a little fat obtained from moderate amounts of low-fat dairy products and meat—is healthiest.

"Choosing to include valuable nutrients in your diet is up to you— a conscious decision you make to reduce your risks of getting cancer."[36]

Vitamins E + C = Overturn Spread of Cancer. Basically, nitrosamines are carcinogens that result from nitrites (a food additive; also found in water from fertilizer runoff) combining with amino acids (from protein foods) in the stomach. These nitrosamines pose a cancer threat. Researchers have found that the combination of vitamin E (400 units daily) with vitamin C (2,000 milligrams daily) could cut nitrosamine formation by as high as 95 percent. This unique duo may well be a much-needed form of nutritional therapy to nip cancer in the bud.[37]

CALLUSES

Symptoms

A sharp stabbing pain on the bottom of your foot indicates the possibility of calluses. About one inch in diameter, they are caused by putting more weight on one part of your foot than another when you walk. You may also develop calluses on your palms, particularly if you do a lot of manual work, or from constant raking of leaves, swinging a tennis racket, rowing a boat, or doing workouts on parallel bars. A callus is a buildup of hard, thick, yellowish skin most often see on the bottom of your foot. The heel is also a common location. Calluses are usually found over diffuse areas on the sole of the foot. Most often, a buildup of callus will result in a "burning" sensation, which hurts more as the day wears on. There is an increase of epidermal cells, causing pressure on the papillae of the skin. The callus is formed by prolonged recurrent pressure and friction. An increase of blood to the area causes an acceleration of cell growth. The additional cells form the callus. Any acutely painful area within a callus requires the immediate attention of your podiatrist, since it might be any one of several other lesions, such as an ulcer, a pseudo-sinus, a hematoma, or a wart. These, too, are essentially symptomatic of some underlying condition, unless you have had an injury to your foot.

Natural Remedies

Elizabeth H. Roberts, D.P.M., a practicing podiatrist in New York City who serves as Professor Emeritus at the New York College of Podiatric Medicine, advises:

"The best protection for callus is a thin piece of moleskin placed directly over the callus, but separated from it by gauze or absorbent cotton. In removing the moleskin each day, be *sure* to hold the skin of your foot taut while you SLOWLY pull the moleskin BACK TOWARDS THE HEEL. Forget all you've ever heard about removing adhesives quickly. Do it SLOWLY and GO BACK TOWARDS THE HEEL. If you don't, you may find a wide, bleeding gash where you've ripped the flesh along with the moleskin.

Overnight Remedies. "It is advisable to leave callus coverings off during the night," says Dr. Roberts, "as well as when you're bathing. This avoids an excessive accumulation of moisture and helps to maintain the healthy tone of the surrounding tissue. (Of course, if your doctor has put a dressing on your callus, it is his or her decision as to whether or not it is to be removed.)

"Do NOT, under any circumstances, indulge in 'bathroom surgery' during which, with razor grasped in one hand, you hold your breath as rigidly as you hold your foot with your other hand. Maybe, to date, you haven't had a blood-bath accident in your self-surgery, but there's always a tomorrow!"[38]

How To Prevent Callus Formation. Dr. Barry H. Block, practicing podiatrist of New York City, tells us, "Calluses are more difficult to prevent than corns are because they are less dependent on your foot structure and the way you walk.

"One way of reducing generalized callus is to wear anti-shearing insoles in your shoes. Two of the best available are Spenco (nitrogen impregnated foam) and PPT (a porometric material). These products are superior to the ordinary 'foam' insoles which are commonly sold in drugstores and supermarkets. Ordinary foam insoles tend to be flimsy, deteriorate rapidly and are relatively ineffective in preventing the frictional shearing force responsible for most calluses.

"For specific calluses, we have the intractable plantar keratoma (IPK), which occurs when one or more of the metatarsals is lower than the others. Metatarsals are the five long bones of the foot. They begin in the middle of the foot and end near the back part of the toes. For these conditions, such as the IPK, orthotic devises are the best prevention.

"Orthotics are custom shoe inserts," says Dr. Block, "which resemble arch supports. Depressions can be built into an orthotic below the area of your callus. These depressions provide space for the dropped bone (usually a metatarsal) to fit in. This prevents your bone from hitting the ground harder than the adjacent bones.

"Orthotics will not correct the underlying structural condition which caused your callus. They will, however, provide accommodative relief. Correction of chronic calluses (particularly IPK's) may require metatarsal surgery."[39]

Cream Softens Callus. Marvin Sandler, D.P.M., a practicing podiatrist of Allentown, Pennsylvania suggests, "Regular use of a good hand cream or lubricating substance can be beneficial for a mild to medium callus. These skin softeners are best rubbed in after a warm bath. Some commercial products designed to 'rub off' callus also have merit."

Can a callus be filed down? Dr. Sandler assures us, "Sometimes. Use pumice stone or a sandpaper file, which can be purchased in a pharmacy. The trick to success with these items is to use them regularly. Not all types of callus will respond, but if you have a callus that is not particularly painful, appropriate use of a pumice stone or callus file can keep the callus under control. **CAREFUL:** If throbbing pain, heat or redness occur, contact your podiatrist immediately because an infection is probably present."[40]

Herbal Soak Is Soothing. To soothe the problem of a lot of callused tissue, you will find relief if you soak your feet in a diluted chamomile tea. Tepid water is helpful. The chamomile herb will soothe and soften the hard skin.

Women and Calluses. Do not mistreat your feet with excessively high-heeled shoes. For the sake of fashion, wear midheight instead of high heels for work. If you must wear high heels (keep to an occasional minimum), look for ones with extra cushioning in the forefoot area. Ask your shoemaker to put extra foam cushioning there. If you have bad calluses on the backs of your heels, avoid open-backed shoes until the area has heeled. And above all, get a proper fit!! Look for natural materials. Avoid friction!! You'll be able to walk . . . callus-free . . . in good health!

CANDIDA ALBICANS

Symptoms

Also known as a vaginal infection, vaginitis, candidiasis. The ailment is caused by an alteration of the normal pH balance of the vagina. When the pH balance changes from its normal, slightly acidic nature to a more alkaline pH, the environment becomes more susceptible to harmful fungi and bacteria. Many vaginitis cases are caused by Candida albicans, a fungus of the yeast family normally found in the skin, mouth, intestinal tract, and vagina. Candida infections, or "yeast infections," occur when the fungus growth becomes uncontrollable owing to a change in the natural pH balance of the vagina. Typical symptoms include intense itching, accompanied by an odorless, white, cheesy discharge. Symptoms do not change from one episode to the next, making it easier to recognize the signs when the infection recurs.

The Infection Spreads. "The incidence of yeast infections is growing due to the increased use of antibiotics and oral contraceptives," cautions Martin Gubernick, M.D., Obestrician and Gynecologist at New York Hospital and Cornell Medical School. "When the normal pH balance of the vagina is disrupted, the Candida albicans fungus multiplies at an alarming rate, causing a vaginal yeast infection. There is severe itching, an odorless white, cottage cheese-like discharge. Nearly 22 million cases are reported each year."

Dr. Gubernick explains that these antibiotics and oral contraceptives "change the pH balance of the vagina to a more alkaline environment, allowing for the growth of harmful bacteria and fungi."

Other Causes. "Additionally, certain factors such as diabetes, and poor eating habits, like diets rich in sugar, cause women to become more susceptible to recurring vaginal yeast infections," adds Dr. Gubernick. Stress and fatigue also contribute to the increase in repeat cases.

Embarrassment of First Time Victims. Most first-time victims of vaginal yeast infections find the experience scary and emotionally upsetting. There is a feeling of being embarrassed, dirty, and victimized. Many are unaware of the cause of the problem or how to treat it effectively. To delay help is to let the condition spread.

How to Prevent Vaginitis from Spreading. Dr. Gubernick offers the following suggestions for preventing the spread of infections:

1. Avoid scratching. It will only irritate the area and cause the infection to spread.

2. Dry the vaginal area after showering, bathing, and swimming. Change out of wet bathing suits or sweaty exercise outfits as soon as possible because the organisms that cause vaginitis thrive in moist conditions.

3. Wipe from front to rear (away from the vagina) following urination and a bowel movement.

4. Wear cotton underwear. Nylon and other synthetic fabrics retain heat and moisture, providing harmful bacteria with a damp environment in which to grow. Choose pantyhose with a cotton crotch.

5. Avoid sexual activity, which can irritate inflamed tissues, and force harmful bacteria into the uterus and fallopian tubes.

6. When menstruating and using any vaginal antifungal medication, avoid using tampons because they may absorb the medication and/or increase inflammation of the vagina.

7. Discuss with your doctor any medications you are presently taking. Certain types, such as antibiotics, can make the vagina more susceptible to infection.

Dr. Gubernick emphasizes, "If you are a first-time sufferer, you have never been told to visit your doctor for a definite diagnosis. I recommend you make a list of your symptoms. Once a definite diagnosis is made, you will feel more comfortable identifying and treating the problem yourself the next time it occurs."[41]

Anti-Yeast Diet Plan. You could be allergic to certain foods that are causing the yeast reaction, says William G. Crook, M.D., specialist in allergy, environmental and preventive medicine of Jackson, Tennessee. "Diet is a key factor in bringing excesses under control." He advises his patients to avoid the following foods for one month, then to reinstate them slowly, once they are feeling better. "But excessive consumption of these foods is not advisable for anyone with a yeast problem," he cautions.

Refined Carbohydrates. Restrict sugar, white flour, white rice.

Sugar-Containing Foods and Beverages. Avoid such products. Do not use maple syrup, molasses or honey.

Yeast Foods. These include yeast breads, rolls, crackers and snack foods containing yeast; many vitamins also have yeast. *Read labels carefully.*

Alcoholic Beverages. Say NO to liquor, beer, wine and cider since all are made with yeast.

Cheeses. The more aged a cheese, the more yeast it contains. You may be able to tolerate ricotta, cottage cheese, cream cheese.

Processed Foods. They are usually high in yeast as compared to non-processed foods. Keep away from bacon, ham, beef jerky, lox, any smoked meats or fish; avoid dried fruits and dried vegetables, which are made with yeast.

Fruits and Fruit Juices. Fruits are rapidly metabolized into sugar which could cause a yeast outbreak. Some fruits may have mold, which worsens the condition. Canned and bottled fruit juices also have a very high yeast content. (After three weeks abstention, if your symptoms subside, try small amounts of whole fruits or freshly squeezed juice to see if they cause reactions.)

Products of Yeast Fermentation. All vinegars and products containing vinegar, such as pickles, mayonnaise, catsup, many salad dressings, barbecue sauce, soy sauce, sour cream, buttermilk. *Note:* You may have yogurt if it is sugar-free, fruit-free because it is fermented with the friendly bacteria lactobacillus instead of yeast.

Coffee, Tea. Subject to mold contamination. Best to avoid or, at least, cut down to a minimum.

Food Additives. Artificial colors, flavors, preservatives may cause a reaction. Again *read labels carefully.*

What is Safe? All vegetables; whole grains, including brown rice, wheat, oats, barley, millet; poultry, seafood, lean meats; unprocessed vegetable oils, especially linseed oil; butter.

With these nutritional adjustments, you will help protect against the occurrence of a vaginal yeast infection.[42]

CASE HISTORY—*Agonizing Itch, Embarrassing Discharge Corrected with Natural Remedies*

In the second half of her menstrual cycle, between ovulation and menses, Susan DeB. developed an intense itch just inside the vagina. This was accompanied by a creamy discharge with a yeasty odor. The area became red and inflamed. She was a nervous wreck because of the agonizing itch. She felt embarrassed about the discharge. When it became unbearable, Susan DeB. went to her allergist. He immediately diagnosed it as Candida albicans and traced its outbreak to her use of antibiotics and oral contraceptives. Adjustments in medications were made. For relief, Susan DeB. followed the preceding Anti-Yeast Diet. It was restrictive, but she was desperate . . . and in three weeks, she was glad since the condition was traced to several food allergies, too. A small adjustment and avoidance of sugar-containing foods helped send candida into remission. The "agony" was relieved, and now she felt wonderful again.

How To Kill Infections with Detergent, Heat. Marjorie Crandall, Ph.D., candida specialist of Torrance, California, suggests better methods of cleansing panties. "Normal laundering does not kill the fungus. Candida albicans survives normal wash-and-dry cycles; once deposited in a woman's panties, there can be another infection."

Dr. Crandall suggests:

- Scrub the crotch of your panties with unscented detergent before putting them into the wash. Avoid bleach or fabric softener, "which irritate delicate skin."
- Boil away the fungus by giving your underpants a hot wash. Or

else, soak them in bleach for 24 hours prior to use to kill the candida. Wash with unscented soap before putting on.

• Kill the fungus with heat—touch your panties with a hot iron.[43]

How to Ease Risks of Infection. Because yeast thrives in a warm, damp environment, keep your vaginal region well ventilated . . . cool and dry. Remove panties when going to sleep. Treat your vaginal area to a cool breath of air.

During the day, your clothes should be comfortably loose. AVOID garments made from plastic, polyester, and leather, since they do not permit full air circulation. Wear fewer layers of clothing. Wear skirts whenever possible, for better ventilation.

Avoid Starch Powders. Starch is food for fungus cultures. Many after-bath powders contain starch, which compounds your problem. Better yet, keep all powders away from your panties!

Keeping Clean with Plain Water. Scented washing products such as soaps, bath salts, bath oils, and shampoo remove your skin's natural protective oils and cause an irritating aftereffect. Plain water and gentle friction will help keep you fresh and clean. A hand-held shower head is most cleansing, since it is directed on the desired area. Using these suggestions, you may be able to build resistance to Candida albicans and enjoy freedom from yeast infections.

CANKER OR COLD SORES

Symptoms

Medically known as *aphthous stomatitis*, they are round or oval lesions, typically in a cluster, that form on the movable tissues in the mouth, usually inside the lips or cheeks but sometimes on or under the tongue. Altogether, the sore is usually less than three-eighths of an inch wide. The lip or cheek at the affected area may swell for about a day. Depending upon the site of the sore, it may hurt to smile, talk, kiss, brush your teeth, eat or drink. Usually, you will experience a single or a few canker sores at a time. They generally heal within two weeks. Severe forms of the sores may leave scars.

A tendency to develop canker sores is often inherited; stress can trigger outbreaks, too. Trauma, such as biting the lip or cheek or scratching the lining of the mouth with a toothbrush, or reactions to certain foods may cause an outbreak. Irritation because of a rough tooth or a poorly-fitting denture can also lead to canker sores. Any constant irritation, including smoking or heavy drinking, and unrelieved tension, as well as food allergy, could lead to eruption of these sores.

Natural Remedies

Jerome Z. Litt, M.D., a dermatologist in Beachwood, Ohio, suggests boosting the body's immune system with bacteria that compete with infectious organisms in canker sores, if they exist. How to do it? Dr. Litt suggests:

1. Eat four tablespoons of yogurt daily, and
2. Drink several glasses of buttermilk a day.

A related remedy is to take L-acidophilus capsules three times a day. Acidophilus is a product of milk-fermenting bacteria and is available in health food stores.

If you have recurrent canker sores, Dr. Litt recommends the following general measures to help prevent attacks:

- Keep your mouth clean.
- Avoid all kinds of nuts and any foods you suspect might be triggering factors.
- No chewing gum, mouthwashes or menthol cigarettes.
- If you are using a fluoridated toothpaste (and who isn't?), switch to a non-fluoridated brand or use salt or baking soda as a substitute.

Tea Bag Remedy. Dr. Litt explains, "You can, however, try treating your canker sores with tea bags at home. The tannic acid in tea, for some unexplained reason, helps heal the sores.

"Directions: Immerse a tea bag in tepid water, remove it, and squeeze out most of the water. Then apply the tea bag directly to the canker sore. You may be pleasantly surprised at the result."

Yogurt Remedy. If you are plagued with recurrent canker sores, Dr. Litt suggests, "I recommend that you eat at least four tablespoonfuls of unflavored yogurt every day. If you do this daily, you may never have a canker sore again!"[44]

TIP: Look for yogurt that contains active cultures of *Lactobacillus acidophilus*.

Vitamin Remedies. Squeeze vitamin E oil from a capsule onto your canker sore. Repeat several times a day to keep the tissue lubricated.

Some people, at the first tingle of a canker sore, find it is helpful to take 500 milligrams of vitamin C with bioflavonoids. Take three times a day for the next five days to help build resistance to this form of immunological breakdown.

Aloe Vera Rinse. This plant has been found to possess healing benefits, especially for inflammation and hurt tissues. You may want to rinse your mouth with aloe vera juice (available in health food stores) several times a day. Aloe contains properties that soothe injuries to the skin and lining tissues, and counteract invading bacteria.

Be Good to Your Mouth. Avoid irritants while you have the condition. Keep away from acidic or spicy foods or drinks until the canker sores heal. You may be able to avoid irritating the sores if you drink such beverages through a straw . . . but do it carefully. Abstain from nuts and popcorn, which can be hurtful. Do not use hard-bristled toothbrushes or other objects that could scrape or cut the lining.

Natural Astringent. Varro E. Tyler, Ph.D., Professor of Pharmacology at Purdue University, in West Lafayette, Indiana, recommends a homemade mouthwash that uses goldenseal root (available at health food stores). Brew a strong tea of this herb and use it as a mouthwash. Or else, make a paste of this herb and apply it directly to your canker sores. "It is antiseptic and astringent," says Dr. Tyler, "and is modestly effective."[45]

❧

CASE HISTORY—*Pesky Canker Sores Respond to Natural Remedies*

Irritating, hurtful canker sores made it uncomfortable for Stuart K. to give talks as a sales manager. He was beset with painful spasms that made him wince while offering a presentation to customers. He was bothered with recurring canker sores because of stress and some food allergies. Stuart K. used chemical-laced mouthwashes, but they brought on more irritation. Eating fresh citrus fruits made him feel a "burning" that was so distressing, he had to give up this important source of vitamins and minerals.

Fortunately, he came across a holistic dentist who suggested he ease up on citrus fruit for a while. He told Stuart K. to take Vitamin C plus bioflavonoids on a daily basis; a total of 1,500 milligrams divided into 500 doses, three times a day. He was also told to eat at least eight tablespoonfuls of unflavored yogurt each day. Then he was to soothe the irritation with daily rinses of aloe vera juice; at night, apply a paste of goldenseal root. And . . . more sleep, less stress! Within nine days, the sores healed! Stuart K. felt "refreshed all over" with a healthy mouth. To prevent recurrence, he continued with this program. These natural remedies helped give him freedom from pesky canker sores.

CARDIOVASCULAR HEALTH

Symptoms

Refers to illnesses of the heart and vascular system. The warning signals of a heart attack include:

- Uncomfortable pressure, fullness, squeezing or pain in the center of the chest lasting two minutes or longer.
- Pain spreading to the shoulders, neck or arms.
- Severe pain, dizziness, fainting, sweating, nausea or shortness of breath.

Not all of these warning symptoms occur in every heart attack. If some of these signs do start to occur, however, do not wait. Seek help immediately. The three major risk factors for cardiovascular illness are cigarette smoking, high blood pressure, and high blood cholesterol. Other risk factors are overweight, diabetes and physical inactivity. While any single risk factor will increase the likelihood of developing heart-related problems, the more risk factors you have, the more concerned you should be about prevention. Your health is improved by giving up smoking, correcting your blood pressure, cholesterol, and overweight. Bring diabetes under control. Keep yourself more active. You'll be giving more lives to your heart!

Natural Remedies

The American Heart Association advises you to eat a "prudent" diet to protect against cardiovascular illness. Based on many such studies, you can eat your way to a healthier heart with these nutritional guidelines as a base for improved health:

1. Reduce total fat—both saturated and unsaturated—to less than 30 percent of your total calories. *Example:* 10 percent saturated,

10 to 15 percent monounsaturated, and the remainder polyunsaturated.

2. Limit calories to achieve and maintain a desirable body weight. Limit "empty" calories from foods that are high in fats and simple sugars.

3. Limit or eliminate your consumption of alcohol.

4. Limit cholesterol-containing foods to no more than 300 milligrams a day—that's six ounces of a cooked, edible portion of meat, fish or poultry.

5. Limit your protein consumption to 15 to 20 percent of total calories.

6. Limit your salt consumption.

7. Increase your intake of foods containing complex carbohydrates and fiber to at least 55 percent of total calories.

Fish Oils—Heart-Saving Catch of the Day. Fish oils contain omega-3 fatty acids, which are believed important in helping to lower fat levels of the blood, thereby improving the health of the heart. This is noted by William Connor, M.D., Chief of Clinical Nutrition at Oregon Health Sciences University, who tells us that eating fish will help diminish risk of heart attack.

"Fish oil has two effects. It lowers triglycerides as well as cholesterol (both are forms of blood fats), and it tends to prevent formation of blood clots." How fast will fish oils work? Dr. Connor adds, "In each of our cases, levels of these blood fats dropped rather rapidly when patients switched from animal and vegetable diets to fish oil. It was observable within two weeks."

Which Fish To Eat? Dr. Connor adds, "People should use this information to eat more fish instead of meat . . . but only fish that is steamed, baked or broiled, Microwave cooking apparently is equally effective, but not fast food (coated and fried) fish. Going to McDonald's for a fish sandwich won't work because it is fried and it has batter on it. Those are the things we do not feel are helpful."[46]

Good sources of Omega-3 fish oils are salmon, mackerel and sardines. Tuna, canned albacore, cod and haddock also have appreciable amounts of this important heart-saving natural food.

Supplements? Be Cautious. Omega-3 fatty acids are available as fish oils in supplements. Be careful—they may cause anticoagulation (bleeding) and a reduced clotting time. Use fish oil capsules with the guidance of your health practitioner. It would make good heart-sense to eat more fish during the week, in any situation. The oils seem to protect the heart from developing abnormal, and often fatal, rhythms after a blockage of blood flow to the heart muscle.

Less Fat-Longer Heart Life. Eating more greens and grains and less (or almost no) animal fat could help ward off heart trouble. Much support for a low-fat vegetarian remedy comes from Dean Ornish, M.D., Assistant Clinical Professor of Medicine at the University of California School of Medicine, San Francisco. Over a period of time, patients who followed a vegetarian diet were able to unclog their arteries and help overcome risks of cardiovascular distress. He found that among those patients with severe heart disease, a low-fat vegetarian diet, stress reduction, and exercise can unplug arteries and reverse heart disease.

Dr. Ornish's supervised program reduces fat to no more than 10 percent of daily calories, and cholesterol intake to 5 milligrams. In a control group, even the patients who took the recommended fat intake of 30 percent of calories or less showed an "artery disease increase."

According to Dr. Ornish, "only a diet almost entirely free of animal fat, oil and cholesterol will significantly lower blood cholesterol levels reliably in just about everyone."

Not Easy . . . But Your Heart Is Worth the Effort. Although Dr. Ornish does not minimize the difficulty for making such changes, he points out, "Once you get started, a diet vibrant with color and rich with flavors and textures of fresh vegetables, beans and pasta, grains and fruit-based desserts could be pleasurable."

Basic Guidelines. The Ornish diet, in addition to limiting fat and excluding oils and animal products (with the exception of non-fat milk and non-fat yogurt), also excludes even non-animal products such as nuts and seeds that are high in fat. It also excludes monosodium glutamate and all stimulants, including coffee. It does allow the consumption of alcohol, but less than two ounces a day. It permits the use of egg white, and allows moderate use of salt and sugar. This plan is also high in important fiber. It does indicate that you can reverse heart disease without drugs, once you take the life style changes far enough.[47]

———————————————— ❧ ————————————————

CASE HISTORY—*Overcomes "Hopeless" Heart Disease with Natural Remedies*

Several heart attacks threatened to make Elaine U. a semi-invalid. The stress of knowing she had an ailing heart compounded the problem.

Even after medications helped reverse atherosclerosis, the slightest "cheating" with fatty foods started the condition again. Elaine U. wanted to overcome her heart trouble, not live with it! A nutritionally-oriented cardiovascular physician prescribed omega-3 fatty acids, and when her arteries became cleansed, he put her on the Dr. Ornish program. In six weeks, after being taken off medication under close supervision, her heart regained its health. Gone were painful symptoms. Tests showed she had given her heart a new life . . . it was possible with stress reduction, more exercise, and a near-vegetarian diet. She could eat egg whites and non-fat milk or yogurt . . . and feel "fat" satisfaction. Elaine U. proclaimed, "These natural remedies gave me a new heart!"

CARPAL TUNNEL SYNDROME

Symptoms

Do you often feel a numbness or tingling in your hand, especially at night? Maybe you experience clumsiness in handling objects. Sometimes you feel a pain that goes up your arm as high as your shoulder. These may be the symptoms of carpal tunnel syndrome. Physicians have traced the condition to a nerve entrapment in the wrist (carpus) and labeled the disorder "carpal tunnel syndrome." A number of medical conditions, such as an underactive thyroid (hypothyroidism), diabetes, rheumatoid arthritis, and gout can give rise to the syndrome.

The syndrome refers to a compression of the median nerve which extends through the wrist and into the thumb, index finger, long finger and part of the ring finger to supply sensation to those digits. The entrapment takes place in a roughly one inch by one half inch wrist opening. The median nerve in each hand shares this carpal tunnel space with nine flexor tendons. Eight go to the fingers and one to the thumb, enabling them to bend.

Causes

One major cause is that of so-called repetitive strain injuries. You keep moving your hand and/or wrist in the same motion, over and over again. An example is that of the assembly line worker, or the garment worker, or laborers using high-power drills or air-operated tools. With the rise of computer video display terminals, these injuries have burgeoned.

The syndrome can result from swelling (edema) in the carpal tunnel as a result of the medical illnesses or from an inflammation (synovitis) in the lining of the tendons caused by exertion upon the wrist by various activities. Since it is the softest structure present in the tunnel, the median nerve can easily become compressed. CAUTION: Pressures within the carpal tunnel reach their highest levels when the wrist is in flexion. Pressure increases symptoms by reducing the blood supply. You may have a referred pain in your forearm and even as far up as your shoulder. The symptoms may arise while you are at the wheel of a car or in some similar sustained activity.

Quick Self-Tests. Do you have the syndrome? Try either or both of these simple, quick self-tests:

1. Tap the palm side of the carpal tunnel with your finger. (A little above your wrist, near your palm.) If the median nerve is compressed, a shooting, tingling pain extends down into your fingers. You may have the syndrome.
2. Rest your elbow on a table. Let your wrist bend completely for one minute. If you feel abnormal sensations in your hand, it could be the syndrome.

To help decrease your chances of carpal tunnel syndrome, try these remedies if you work with terminals or some other working apparatus:

- Keep your computer keyboard low. Put it in your lap if you must. Make sure the top of your display screen is at eye-level. Use a chair of proper height.
- Take frequent breaks from repetitive tasks.
- Avoid bending your wrists. Use bent-handled scissors, knifes, or pliers, for instance. Keep your wrists in a neutral position.
- Try to keep hands warm while you work. Wear gloves, if necessary.

Vitamin B_6 Eases Symptoms. John Ellis, M.D., a surgeon and family practitioner in Mount Pleasant Texas, has found that vitamin B_6 on a daily basis can ease symptoms of this disorder. He believes that "carpal tunnel syndrome is caused by a deficiency, pure and simple. In a high percentage of cases, the patients are deficient in vitamin B_6." He prescribes a daily dose of 50 milligrams and found that this relieved the symptoms nearly every time. "Sometimes patients responded rapidly; in other cases, they took six or even twelve weeks to improve. These patients frequently had swollen hands and fingers. Vitamin B_6 or pyridoxine, usually relieved this as well." He adds, "During the time you take the vitamin, the symptoms gradually begin to subside. You have to be patient. You will notice a decided difference in your hands and fingers. The numbness, tingling, stiffness and pain in your hand subsides."

Suppose you discontinue the vitamin? Dr. Ellis says, 'A number of people have a recurrence of carpal tunnel syndrome when they stop taking the vitamin." He emphasizes the need for being patient. The vitamin does more than merely activate existing B_6-dependent enzymes, a process that takes only a few days. "Vitamin B_6 must also increase the total number of enzyme molecules, a process called enzyme induction. So . . . don't give up!"[48]

Change Sleeping Position. The syndrome is worse at night because carpal tunnel tissues swell if you sleep with limp, curled wrists. The **only** way to relieve numbness and pain is to change your sleeping posture. Bring your hand **lower** than your heart. Your arm must be straight down from your shoulder. Keep a straight elbow, straight wrist.

Use A Plastic Wrist Brace. To help maintain a comfortable straight elbow and straight wrist, put on a plastic brace that is laced gently and positioned with velcro fasteners. It eases discomfort and relieves numbing pain. The brace is available at surgical supply shops. Wear it during the day and while you sleep to minimize strain to your wrist.

Correct the Tools You Use. Select scissors with angled blades that curve toward your thumb when you hold them so you keep your wrist straight. Other tools should have a big rubber handle instead of a hard, slippery plastic one. Select pliers and other tools engineered to keep your hand straight when it is doing its work, instead of shifting to the right or left or up and down. You can custom fit a tool handle by building it up with bathroom caulking.

Round and Round You Go! Feel a warning tingle? Try a circle exercise. Move your hands around in gentle circles for three minutes. You will exercise all wrist muscles, improve circulation, take your wrist out of the bent position that brings on the syndrome. Repeat at least six times throughout the day.

Arms Go Up . . . Higher and Higher. Take a break from your workstation before it breaks you! Raise both arms over your head. Rotate your arms and wrists simultaneously. Do this for three minutes. You will ease stress and promote more flexibility. Repeat at least six times throughout the day.

Rotate Your Head. Place hands on a table and rotate your head for about three minutes. Move backward and forward, then from one side to the other. Look over your right shoulder, over your left shoulder. Do this for two minutes. Repeat six times throughout the day.

Your purpose is to include these simple exercises in your daily schedule to keep your muscles and tendons loose and flexible.

Ice That Pain. Tendonitis (inflammation of tendons) responds well to an ice bath or ice rub. Do the same for your carpal tunnel syndrome. An ice pack helps cool and reduce that swelling. **CAREFUL:** Do not use heat, which increases swelling.

Squeeze Your Pain. Shake hands with yourself. Push one palm against the other. Make a bridge of both of your hands and press against each other. Stretch your fingers all the way back and hold. Repeat several times. The pain and tingling feeling is relieved.

Carrying Tips. Whatever you carry, the handle should have a fit that grips. If too small, use rubberized tubing or tape. Too large a grip? Get a different handle.

If your wrist is repeatedly flexed, the pressure builds up. You could be wringing wet laundry by hand, sweeping with a broom, even peeling or shelling food. You could be behind the wheel of a truck, a pneumatic-hammer worker. Musicians, especially piano players with a chair too low, using crooked wrists, have the problem. Improve position with a higher chair, using straight wrists to minimize pain. Or a carpenter, racquetball player, gymnast, supermarket checker, knitter . . . or any task that calls for repetitive movements of your wrists. Protect yourself against this syndrome with these natural remedies. And remember to try to keep your hands and wrists as straight as possible. You may feel it strange when working at a keyboard or driving, but with practice, you'll be able to manage it . . . and your wrists will be all the happier for it. So will you!

CHLAMYDIA

Symptoms

One of the most common of sexually transmitted diseases, chlamydia is a bacterial infection affecting men and women. Men may notice a discharge from the penis and have a persistent urge to urinate even though it is hurtful. Women may experience a vaginal discharge, with some burning during urination. Chlamydial infections are easily confused with gonorrhea because the symptoms of both diseases are similar, and they often occur together. Many doctors recommend that all persons who have more than one sex partner, and especially women under age 35, be tested for chlamydial infection each year. Rapid diagnostic tests use sophisticated techniques and a dye to detect the bacterium (*Chlamydia trachomatis*); they can be performed during a routine checkup and results are available within 30 minutes.

Untreated, Chlamydia can cause pain, fever, miscarriage, and infertility in women. Infants born to infected women can develop eye infections and pneumonia. The infection is also associated with premature labor and low birth weight. In men, chlamydia may lead to epididymitis, a serious and painful disease of the testicles. It rarely causes sterility in males.

Natural Remedies

The most important remedy is to have a regular examination that includes a test for this ailment. Any sexually active woman, especially if she is in her earlier years and takes birth control pills, should have the test. **DANGER:** Chlamydia blocks or destroys the female's fallopian tubes, causing sterility or endangering pregnancy as well as being potentially life threatening to the mother in tubal pregnancies. It also causes pelvic inflammatory disease.

Barrier Contraceptive. Researchers note that women who use a diaphragm, condom or cervical cap with a spermicide have much less of a risk of suffering from tubal infertility than users of non-barrier methods of contraception. One reason: pelvic inflammatory disease brought on by chlamydia can cause injury to the fallopian tubes. Barrier contraceptives help prevent this hurt by stopping infections from reaching the tubes.[49]

Regular Tests. It is important that if you are diagnosed as having a chlamydial infection, your partner is also treated. Otherwise, there is a chance of being reinfected. If you have urinary or cervical infections that recur, or your partner has recently developed a urinary tract infection, you may have the problem of chlamydia.

CHOLESTEROL

Symptoms

An invisible risk because there are no outward symptoms! Cholesterol is a fatty, wax-like substance found naturally in all body cells. It is used by your body to build cells and make hormones; it also aids in food digestion. Your liver can manufacture all the cholesterol your body needs. But cholesterol also comes from animal foods such as eggs, fatty meats, butter and whole milk. You may have an overload of cholesterol, and this could cause danger.

Increase Risk of Heart Attack. Excess cholesterol in the blood may collect in fatty streaks along the inner linings of the arteries. These fatty deposits, along with clotted blood and scar tissue, slowly build up to form fibrous plaque. This process is called atherosclerosis or hardening of the arteries. DANGER: The artery wall thickens and becomes less flexible, while the arterial opening narrows and hampers the normal blood flow. Eventually, the artery may become entirely blocked. If this artery feeds the brain, a stroke may result. If the artery connects to the heart, a heart attack may occur. In other areas of the body, the narrowed or clogged artery may cause injury to other tissues.

"Good" Versus "Bad" Cholesterol. High-density lipoprotein (HDL) is the "good" cholesterol because it helps remove excess cholesterol from the blood. Low-density lipoprotein (LDL) is the "bad" cholesterol because high levels lead to a build-up of cholesterol in the artery walls.

What Are Desirable Cholesterol Levels? The chart below defines cholesterol risk levels for different age groups.

Age	Average Blood Cholesterol mg/dl	Moderate Risk	High Risk
20–29	180–199	200–219	220+
30–39	200–219	220–239	240+
40+	200–239	240–259	260+

Source: National Institutes of Health/National Heart, Lung and Blood Institute

When having your cholesterol level checked, ask your practitioner to test it along with your LDL and HDL levels. Each check involves a simple blood test. A high ratio of LDL to HDL may signal the need for correction, even if your overall cholesterol is low. Women, on average, have higher levels of HDL than men, which may be one reason for their lower incidence of heart disease. For those people whose families have a history of high blood cholesterol or coronary heart disease, regular testing should begin around age 20. *Note:* If you have a level over 200, you should immediately start programs to control an overload of cholesterol.

Natural Remedies

Your first program is to limit cholesterol intake to 250–300 milligrams a day. Reduce fat intake to 30 percent of total calories. Cut saturated fat intake to 10 percent of total calories by replacing them with polyunsaturated and monounsaturated fats. If weight loss is needed, total caloric intake should be reduced.

Tips to Reduce Fats and Cholesterol. Follow these remedies:

- Eat less butter, margarine, oil and other fats overall; eat fewer fried foods.
- Choose fish, poultry and lean cuts of meat; limit or avoid sausage, bacon and processed luncheon meats.
- Trim fat from meats before cooking; remove skin from poultry before eating.
- Limit or avoid organ meats such as liver, kidney or sweetbreads.
- Use skim or low-fat or non-fat milk and milk products including cheese and yogurt; choose ice milk over ice cream.
- Eat more high-fiber foods such as fruits, vegetables, whole grains and cereals to replace high-fat foods.
- Avoid baked goods made with lard, coconut oil, palm oil or shortening.
- Use fewer egg yolks, more egg whites in cooking.

Give Up Smoking. Carbon monoxide in the blood of smokers also damages artery walls, increasing susceptibility to plaque build-up. Keep away from those who smoke since the "sidestream" can be as potent as if you are smoking!

Omega-3's Control Cholesterol. Omega-3's are a type of polyunsaturated fatty acid found in fish. The unique structure of the omega-3 fatty acid has been shown to influence how your body metabolizes fat. These fish oils may also reduce platelet stickiness, actually thinning your blood. *Sources:* salmon, albacore tuna, and mackerel. Try substituting fish for red meat in your diet three times a week.

Fiber Lowers Cholesterol. Fiber is the carbohydrate that is not digested and does not provide nutrients. But it functions by helping to "wash out" cholesterol. There are *two* types of fiber:

1. *Insoluble fiber* provides bulk and aids in the movement of food and water through your intestine. Recommended for treatment of constipation and diverticular disease. Sources: whole wheat, corn, vegetables.

2. *Soluble fiber* ferments in the intestine to form substances that prevent the liver from producing cholesterol. These substances attach to bile acids—the products of cholesterol metabolism— and remove them from the body through elimination. Sources: oats, legumes (dried beans, peas, lentils), guar gum, psyllium seeds, some fruits and vegetables.

Control Cholesterol with Soluble Fibers. James W. Anderson, M.D., Professor of Medicine and Clinical Nutrition at the University of Kentucky in Lexington has found that by boosting the intake of soluble fiber-rich foods, cholesterol levels can be controlled and reduced. "This type of fiber reduces the LDL cholesterol, or the undesirable kind. It does not interfere with the HDL cholesterol, the favorable kind." Dr. Anderson recommends boosting intake of more legumes and grains to help offset cholesterol overload.

Simple Daily Plan. "Most people can lower cholesterol by eating 2/3 cup of oat bran cereal or one cup of beans per day," says Dr. Anderson. "I also recommend about six grams of soluble fiber per day for most people. You can get that from one half cup of oat bran cereal or one cup of beans."[50]

Niacin (Vitamin B_3) And Cholesterol. William E. Connor, M.D., Professor of Clinical Medicine, Chief of Endocrinology and Clinical Nutrition at Oregon Health Sciences University, in Portland, has found that niacin can be part of an effective cholesterol-lowering program. It should be used under supervision because the doses required are high and could cause reactions such as flushing of the skin. If taken throughout the day in smaller doses, it would prove to be beneficial [51]

Fitness Controls Cholesterol. Don't just sit there with nutritional remedies. Stimulate your metabolism with regular exercise, such as walking, doctor-approved jogging. More physical activity helps raise your "good" HDL cholesterol and lower your "bad" LDL cholesterol. This ratio improves your immunity against cardiovascular distress. Schedule 60 minutes daily of brisk exercise as part of your cholesterol control program. It could be as important as nutrition . . . perhaps more so!

CASE HISTORY—*Brings Down Cholesterol with Food and Fitness*

A sedentary lifestyle gave Norman W. an unusually high cholesterol reading. He had atherosclerosis, traced to fatty foods. He was overweight. His cholesterol was 240. His health specialist prescribed a daily walking program together with more "get up and go," instead of sitting so much. He was put on more oat bran cereal and muffins and less (much less) fatty foods. Seafood appeared three times a week. In three months, he had cleaner arteries, a healthier cholesterol of 195, a trimmer figure . . . and hope for a longer lifeline!!

CHRONIC FATIGUE SYNDROME OR EPSTEIN-BARR VIRUS

Symptoms

Chronic fatigue syndrome, also known as CFS, is debilitating and involves a group of related symptoms such as: headache, sore throat, fever, weakness, lymph node pain, muscle and joint pain, memory loss, and difficulty in concentrating. In some persons, the symptoms of CFS follow an illness resembling influenza or other non-specific acute viral disease. In many, CFS develops gradually, with no detectable cause. There is a link between CFS and the Epstein-Barr virus (EBV), which causes similar symptoms. Although EBV alone is not necessarily the culprit, there is a connection. Many people have mood swings or panic attacks. Most develop a low-grade dementia. Sleep disturbances are common, as are vision problems. Why does it happen? A belief is that it is caused by an immunological defect in which the immune system goes into overdrive fighting off infection and producing substances that make the body feel sicker. Stress, environmental toxins, and virus exposure may spark the disorder or cause eruption of dormant symptoms.

Natural Remedies

Basically, you are advised to eat properly, get plenty of rest, avoid stress. A diet free of preservatives, food dyes and caffeine, and low in fats, salt and sugar is most helpful. To rebuild your weakened immune system, restructure your lifestyle to do the following:

- A good night's sleep is mandatory. Throughout the day, take relaxation breaks and ease up on stress.
- Improve your eating. Adequate amounts of vitamins and minerals can make a difference. Minimize intake of fat and sugar. Avoid caffeine!
- Exercise each day is invigorating. Too fatigued? Try stretching. Walking in place. Going up the stairs . . . one or two flights if it is too tiring to do more. Avoid overexertion, but also avoid being too sedentary. You will **not** recover by remaining in bed! You could become an invalid! Keep yourself active.
- You have a certain amount of energy. Don't draw out more than you have or you could go bankrupt! Instead, schedule your activities . . . a little at a time. Use your energy carefully. You'll last much longer.
- Anticipate problems and their solutions. Whenever you plan an activity, preview potential problems. Have alternatives ready if problems arise. Rehearse what you would do if . . . your car broke down on the highway . . . overwhelming fatigue hits while you are shopping . . . you miss connections while traveling. Taking risks can be stressful, but careful pre-planning and preparation will reduce stress and fatigue and make activities more enjoyable.
- Know your limitations. You could be caught in the grip of fatigue. Delay unnecessary tasks. Delegate the others. Use relaxation techniques, pamper yourself, listen to music, light some scented candles, take an herbal-fragrance bath, read a funny book (you need more laughter!). Do **NOT** feel sorry for yourself! An important concept in stress management is to accept what you cannot change instead of constantly being frustrated over situations beyond your control. Have reasonable expectations for yourself and for others.

Are You Sick and Tired of Feeling Sick and Tired? Don't just blame yourself or others and hide under your blankets! Do something to improve your situation. Make rest periods a high priority. Schedule them before and after any activity on your calendar. Is there a time of day when you are likely to be at your best? Set aside that time for your most demanding activities. Consolidate and simplify tasks. When cooking, double the recipe and freeze part for later. Typing (computer, word processor, typewriter) uses less energy than handwriting. Organize your household by keeping all equipment necessary for any task together in one area. **TIP:** Sit whenever possible to conserve energy. Having a high stool to work at the kitchen counter can reduce fatigue and pain. Put dishes on an inexpensive wheeled cart or table, and you save steps and energy when setting the table.

Divide more difficult tasks into smaller parts. Take frequent rest breaks. Even on your best days, pace yourself. Set small short-term goals for yourself. Try to think of tasks that are compatible with your lowest energy level, such as writing a note to someone special, paying a bill, working on a hobby. Do these when you have less stamina. You'll feel good knowing that you began a project in spite of your limitations. Never feel guilty for not getting as much done as you think you should.

Be Wary of Stress. Both excess stress and depression can disrupt your body's hormonal balance and immune system, rendering you more susceptible to CFS infection. Many such patients have well-defined allergies, which could reflect a hypersensitive immune system. Try not to push yourself to the point of collapse. Readjust your schedules and expectations of accomplishments. Allow extra time to get things done. You'll help build resistance to the symptoms of this chronic fatigue ailment . . . and enjoy life all the more!

COLDS

Symptoms

Colds are viral infections of the cells that line the nose and throat (the nasopharynx or upper respiratory tract). During a cold, virus particles penetrate the mucosal blanket and insert their material into the nasopharyngeal cells. In a short time, there is a release of particles, which spreads the cold. The first symptom is usually a sore throat. Then the nose becomes congested and runny. This ailment is an upper respiratory viral infection, with the characteristic symptoms of feeling nasal congestion and discharge, headache and low-grade fever. Inflamed membranes in the nose and throat may cause discomfort day and night, making normal life (including sleep) difficult. You want help!

Natural Remedies

Ira W. Gabrielson, M.D., M.P.H., Professor and Chairman of the Department of Community and Preventive Medicine at the Medical College of Pennsylvania, in Philadelphia tells us, "There are many things we can do during the harsh winter months that will help ward off colds and other cold problems." Dr. Gabrielson offers this set of cold-healing natural remedies:

1. *Wash Your Hands.* Believe it or not, a cold virus has to be handed to you by a cold sufferer to give you a cold; it is not particularly infectious when it comes to you via a sneeze or a cough, but it is a good idea not to get in the way! The reason? Simple: If you get a virus on your hands, poke into your nose—bang—the cold virus finds a new home. It makes good sense not to pick your nose. Dispose of soiled tissues. Wash your hands.

2. *Humidify Your House.* During the winter, many heating systems keep home environments too dry. This can dry out the moist lining of the nasal membranes and respiratory passages. Humidifiers, either run in the bedroom at night or attached to the house's central heating system, help add moisture to the dry air in the house during the harsh winter months. **TIP:** Keep your thermostat at 68°F. When your home is cooler, air can hold and retain more moisture.

3. *Avoid Tobacco Smoke.* The nicotine and tars in tobacco smoke dry and irritate the lining of the nasal membranes and respiratory passages, much in the same way as dry indoor air, and with the same penalties.

4. *Outer Garments.* Hat, gloves, and boots are important to wear during the frigid, windy days of winter. Since about 17 percent of your body heat goes through your head, you should wear a hat. Boots or rubbers are good because they keep you dry. Gloves or mittens help prevent cracked, rough and reddened hands.

5. *Care of Your Skin.* To keep moisture in your skin, use creams such as petroleum jelly. A light coat is helpful. **TIP:** After washing your hands, apply hand lotion while your skin is still damp. It retains moisture better when slightly wet.[52]

How Elderly Can Beat the Common Cold. Cold weather gives us all a nip, but folks over 60 are more susceptible to the chill. People with diabetes or arterial sclerosis are more vulnerable to the cold. You are cautioned to spend as little time as possible outdoors on a very cold day.

More cold enters through your feet, hands, head and face openings. **TIP:** Two pairs of socks or stockings, sheepskin-lined gloves, hat that covers the ears, and scarf over the mouth will be helpful. **CAUTION:** Do not rush out into the cold immediately after eating. It is a good idea to have a wholesome meal from 30 minutes to one hour before going out. The food, which has had a chance to digest, then acts as fuel to help keep your body warm.

Vitamin C to the Rescue. Vitamin C stimulates production of interferon; it boosts the ability of your thymus gland to produce T-cells, which enhances your immune system to overcome colds. Vitamin C also improves your cold-fighting power of bacterial phagocytosis; that is, the ability of phagocytes to destroy infectious bacteria. In various studies, 1,000 to 3,000 grams of vitamin C daily has helped overturn the severity of the common cold. The symptoms are also eased because Vitamin C acts as an internal cleanser, sweeping up the virus debris and strengthening your resistance to infection.

Warm Up with Wool. Insulate yourself with a fuzzy, thick fabric to trap more air than a thin, smooth one. Wool is helpful because it is thick, it has a kinky, scaly fiber that traps air to keep you warm. Wool also absorbs perspiration so your body does not lose heat evaporating it.

Synthetic Fabrics Are Protective. Acrylics, polyesters, acetates and tri-acetates are good insulators because the fibers can be crimped like wool to provide good air-trapping qualities. They are resilient, retaining original thickness very well. CAUTION: They do not always absorb perspiration as well as natural fibers; thus, valuable body heat is lost evaporating moisture on the skin. TIP: Rayon, which is made from wool or cotton, does, however, absorb perspiration efficiently.

Easing Symptoms of Your Cold. To manage your cold, suggested natural remedies include:

- Try a salt water gargle to ease your sore throat. About ¼ teaspoon of salt to eight ounces of water will do the trick.
- Saline nose drops (also ¼ teaspoon of salt to eight ounces of water) helps clear your congested nasal passages.
- Lots and lots of fluids. They will ease your dry throat and promote inner cleansing.
- Time-honored chicken soup is comforting as would be most hot beverages. The taste and aroma, as well as the inhalation of the vapor of chicken soup makes you feel very good. There is a simultaneous increase of the flow of nasal secretions and this eases congestion. Herbal tea with honey is also comforting.
- A sore nose and lips can often be eased with a light application of petroleum jelly or lotion.

- Coughing serves a useful purpose by clearing secretions from your throat. Unless approved by your health practitioner, cough suppressants should not be used for wet productive coughs. Instead, try comfortably hot beverages.
- Get extra rest after work. It is not necessary to stay home if you feel well enough to accomplish something, providing you do not weaken yourself and do not needlessly expose others.

Relax and Free Yourself from Stress. Emotional upset and unrelieved stress can weaken your immune system, depress your resistance and make you more vulnerable to colds, among other ailments. Adjust your attitude. Minimize stress. Mobilize your immune system. Take a "visualization break," and relax quietly in a quiet room. Picture yourself being cleansed. A multitude of scrubbers are sweeping up and detoxifying your congested areas and cleansing away the debris. The relaxation is helpful in stimulating your immune system to cast out the infection.

Garlic Is a Natural Antibiotic. Ingredients in garlic help detoxify your system and "knock out" harmful invaders. If you take only one clove of garlic daily, you will be able to kill germs more rapidly and overcome cold symptoms all the more quickly. **TIP:** A clove of garlic every day of the year is a great way to strengthen your immune system to resist onset of infections.

Two Herbs that Heal Colds. Goldenseal revitalizes your liver to help cleanse your system and filter out infectious wastes. Goldenseal also helps invigorate and strengthen the weakened nasal mucous membranes. Echinacea functions as a cleanser of your lymph and blood glands; it promotes the distribution of infection-fighting antibodies and removes toxic substances. *How To Use:* Health stores and herbal outlets have these two herbs in the form of easy-to-use capsules. One or two capsules of each herb taken with a warm beverage will start the healing process.

Steam Away Your Congestion. Try a steamy shower for about 15 minutes but not to the point of exhaustion. Perspiring is a great way to cleanse away infection. *Alternate:* Heat a pot of water (or teakettle) to boiling on your stove. Turn off the flame. Drape a thick towel as a tent over your head and the pot. Slowly i–n–h–a–l–e the steam. Breathe in. Breathe out. Keep up this remedy until the steam subsides. You will feel relief for your nasal congestion as well as your cough because of the soothing moisture. Try the remedy twice a day for comfortable relief.

If You Stay at Home. The California Medical Association suggests, "A typical common cold will last three to four days. A mild secondary bacterial infection often prolongs this to a week or longer. You should rest in a room with adequate moisture and a comfortable temperature. Your body can best heal itself if it is neither too hot nor too cold. A vaporizer or humidifier can be used to increase moisture. Your nose functions best with the humidity at 70 percent. If your cold lasts more than seven days or if you develop a fever higher than 102°F, an ear infection, laryngitis or bronchitis, see your health practitioner."[53]

COLITIS

Symptoms

An inflammation of the colon and/or rectum could cause an excessive desire to eliminate; there are mild cramps of the lower abdomen along with intermittent diarrhea that passes mucus and blood. *Ulcerative colitis* is the more complete name of this ailment in which the lining of the colon (large bowel) and rectum become inflamed. When this happens, the bowel tries to empty itself frequently, causing diarrhea. As cells on the surface of the lining of the colon die and slough off, ulcers (tiny open sores) form, causing mucus and bleeding. There may be loss of appetite, unnatural weight loss, anemia and arthritis-like pain.

Natural Remedies

You may have a sensitivity to certain foods or food products. If you experience outbreaks after taking such items, eliminate them, to see if you have an allergy.

Control Fiber Intake. Fiber tends to increase stool volume and bloats the bowel, causing irritation of the colon. You may find relief if you keep fiber intake to a minimum. Limit raw fruits and vegetables as well as grains, seeds, nuts, legumes. ((*Note*: Because these foods are good sources of vitamins B complex and C, it would be wise to replace these lost nutrients with a multi-vitamin supplement containing the RDA.) After the diarrhea has eased off, gradually bring back the raw foods and the other fiber-rich foods. Do it slowly!

Skip Dairy Products. For ulcerative colitis, dairy products can be upsetting. Omit them if you observe they cause reactions. (*Note*: Dairy foods offer good sources of dietary calcium so replace with a 1000 milli-gram supplement of calcium in the form of calcium carbonate. Take

500 milligrams at noontime, another 500 at night.) Gradually bring back dairy foods as you recover.

Stay Away from Carbonated and/or Iced Drinks. When you shock your system with these beverages, they trigger excessive activity of the intestinal walls and worsen your diarrhea.

Divide Meals Throughout the Day. You will speed up healing and be less likely to distend your bowel if you schedule smaller, more frequent meals throughout the day. Do not overload your stomach!

Bland Foods Soothe Your Digestive System. Foods should be mild or bland so that you do not irritate your intestinal lining or cause diarrhea.

Calm Your Colon. Tension can react upon your colon and cause unrest, leading to colitis, among other ailments. Practice daily relaxation programs. Avoid disputes or heated arguments. A calm and tranquil life-style will help speed up healing of your colon . . . and the rest of your body, too.

Pectin Is Helpful. Researchers at the University of Pennsylvania feel that the colon can atrophy (weaken) without fiber. They gave pectin—a water-soluble form of fiber—to test subjects. Those receiving pectin had a significant reduction in the degree of bowel injury from colitis. The researchers theorize that pectin may help promote the normal bacterial growth in the colon and help absorb acetic acid . . . without producing unwanted fecal bulk. Pectin is available as a supplement and may be used with the guidance of your health practitioner.[54]

Nutritional Remedies

Sue Rodwell Williams, R.D., Ph.D., of the University of California, Berkeley, suggests, "The dietary treatment for ulcerative colitis may be accompanied by bed rest and psychotherapy. In the acute stage, a liquid diet may be given. The diet following the acute stage may be the minimum-residue diet; as the patient improves, the low-residue diet may be given.

"As soon as safety allows, a bland high-protein, high-calorie diet may be given, according to the physician's directions. The greater selection of foods serves to improve the patient's morale.

"The diet should also be high in vitamins and minerals," says Dr. Williams. "In addition to vitamins in the diet, vitamin supplements, especially vitamin B complex, should be given in double the normal amounts. Large amounts of vitamins are needed because of lack of absorption.

The amount of protein should be high because of the amount of protein lost in the wastes and through hemorrhage. The diet should be low in fat; the only fats used should be butter and cream. Supplementary iron should also be given, since anemia is frequently found in ulcerative colitis. Milk is usually not tolerated well. If the patient cannot take milk, a calcium supplement should be given.

"The patient probably should be eating three meals a day and have between-meal feedings. Adequate fluids must be taken in the amount of 6 to 8 glasses daily. Nervous strain, emotional tension and fatigue should be avoided."[55]

CASE HISTORY—*Corrects Embarrassing and "Crippling" Colitis with Nutritional Remedies*

Office supervisor Joan H. felt like an invalid with her colitis. "Almost crippled!" she declared because her bouts with diarrhea made her housebound. If she kept taking more sick leave, she would lose her lucrative position. Medications made her dizzy. She resisted surgery. Yet she could not go on with this ailment. She sought help from a nutritional chiropractor who put her on a strict nutritional program—less fiber, less dairy, several short meals throughout the day, and no tension! Being relaxed would help her nutritional buildup! She followed this program, took the recommended supplements, and gradually felt her symptoms easing. She also took several pectin tablets daily to further strengthen her colon. Joan H. was soon able to do more than report to work daily . . . she could work overtime. Symptoms? They disappeared. Her immune system had transformed her from a "cripple" to a "careerist" as she overcame "hopeless" colitis!!

CONSTIPATION

Symptoms

A condition in which bowel movements are hard and passed with discomfort, difficulty or pain. The muscles of the colon must work harder to expel resistant wastes out of the body. Constipation is a symptom, not a disease. It is defined as a decrease in the frequency of bowel movements, accompanied by prolonged or difficult passage of waste. There is no accepted rule for the correct number of daily or weekly bowel movements.

"Regularity" may be a twice-daily bowel movement for some or two bowel movements a week for others. Lengthy constipation does call for help.

Natural Remedies

The National Institutes of Health suggests you try these remedies:

1. Eat more fresh fruits and vegetables, either cooked or raw, and more whole-grain cereals and breads. Dried fruits such as apricots, prunes and figs are especially high in fiber. Try to cut back on highly processed foods (such as sweets) and foods high in fat.

2. Drink plenty of liquids (one to two quarts daily) unless you have heart, circulatory or kidney problems. **CAUTION:** Be aware that some people become constipated from drinking large quantities of milk.

3. Some doctors recommend adding *small* amounts of unprocessed bran (also known as "miller's bran") to baked goods, cereals and fruits as a way of increasing the fiber content of your diet. If you *do* use unprocessed bran, remember that some people suffer from bloating and gas for several weeks after adding bran to their diet. All changes should be made slowly, to allow the digestive system to adapt.

4. Stay active. Even taking a brisk walk after dinner can help tone your muscles.

5. Try to develop a regular bowel habit. If you have had problems with constipation, attempt to have a bowel movement shortly after breakfast or dinner.

6. Avoid taking laxatives if at all possible. Although they will usually relieve the constipation, you can quickly come to depend on them and the natural muscle actions required for elimination will be impaired.

7. Limit your intake of antacids, as some can cause constipation as well as other health problems.

8. Above all, do not expect to have a bowel movement every day or even every other day. "Regularity" differs from person to person. If your bowel movements are usually painless and occur regularly (whether the pattern is three times a day or two times each week), then you are probably not constipated.[56]

Figs: Natural Laxative. Fresh figs are a powerhouse of ingredients that will help stimulate sluggish muscle. California figs are especially beneficial. One-half cup offers close to 17 grams, much more than any of the other common fruits said to be high in fiber. When you take one-half cup of figs with a fruit juice, you help bulk waste and move it through the colon more easily and rapidly. Figs are also rich in vitamins and minerals, notably calcium! Figs are a much more concentrated source of fiber than traditional grains, so aim for a balance.

Answer the Call of Nature. Toilet train yourself and heed the call. Otherwise, you may develop encroaching constipation. The most natural time is after a meal so plan ahead. Condition your colon to act as Nature intended.

Relax . . . Take It Easy. Stress can give you a feeling of tightness. If stress is causing your constipation, take time to relax. Listen to soothing music. Try reading relaxation books. Never strain! You risk giving yourself anal fissures or hemorrhoids. You could lower your heartbeat and raise your blood pressure. Easy does it!

Yogurt Helps Establish Regularity. Yogurt contains *Lactobacillus acidophilus*, a bacterial strain that improves the presence of beneficial bacteria in the intestines. (It simultaneously lowers cholesterol absorption.)

Morning Regularity Tonic. To start off the day feeling better, try this Morning Regularity Tonic. In a glass of freshly boiled water, add the juice of one-half lemon and two teaspoons of honey. Stir and sip slowly. This Tonic helps produce morning regularity.

Hints, Tips, Suggestions. Roughage or fiber is important in overcoming constipation. Increase these high-fiber foods: whole grains, cabbage, cauliflower, asparagus, tomatoes, onions, and legumes; also apples, pears, oranges, grapes, figs, raisins, and prunes. In the morning, eat two small whole apples (cored and seeded, of course), and follow with one or two glasses of freshly boiled water to which you add a teaspoon of honey. This program works for many of the most stubborn cases. CAREFUL: Any diet that depends on only one food—such as only dairy foods or eating just green vegetables—can be constipating.

Exercise Promotes Regularity. Rhythmic leg movements, such as those involved in walking, running, biking, dancing or swimming are especially good for stimulating bowel action. Regular physical activity helps relieve tensions that otherwise inhibit the action of the bowel muscles and strengthens the muscles of the abdomen and pelvis, which aid the functioning of the digestive tract. CAREFUL: Early-morning exercisers may find that it helps to have a bowel movement before the daily exercise session, lest they develop the urge at an inconvenient moment. Ideally, you should exercise once a day and a minimum of five times a week.

Tasty Sources of Fiber. You have a good selection from whole grain products, such as crackers, bran muffins, brown rye, oatmeal, pumpernickel, bran and corn breads, whole wheat English muffins and bagels. Try breakfast cereals, such as bran cereals, shredded wheat, whole grain or whole wheat flaked cereals, and others that list dietary fiber content on the package. (Avoid those made with sugar, salt and chemicals!) Fiber, or roughage, represents plant matter that the human digestive tract cannot process. All have a natural laxative effect because they add bulk and absorb and hold on to water, making the stool softer and easier to pass as well as better able to stimulate the muscular action of the colon.

Constipation is no joke. It can be hurtful. The cause is often easy to identify and correct . . . so you can enjoy regularity . . . and happier health.

CORNS

Symptoms

Corns are a common cause of foot pain. They are thickenings of the outer layers of the skin, caused by pressure and/or friction of the skin rubbing against underlying bony areas when walking. If the first signs of soreness are ignored, corns rise up as Nature's attempt to protect sensitive areas. Most corns are dense and form on the toes. Abnormal stresses such as friction stimulate the skin to grow faster than the body can shed it, giving rise to the formation of corns. This friction generally occurs when the skin finds itself squeezed between the shoe on the outside and a foot bone on the inside. Often an underlying bursa (balloon-like sac that surrounds a joint and fills with fluids in response to joint irritation) is associated with a corn.

There is a sound basis for the old wives' tale that people with corns can predict an approaching storm. When the barometer drops, the atmospheric pressure decreases. This causes the fluid in the bursa below a corn to expand, thus making the corn even more hurtful. Do your corns hurt more during inclement weather? Do you feel pain when the sides of your corn are squeezed? You most likely have an inflamed bursa underneath your corn.

Natural Remedies

Do **not** attempt self-treatment if you have such conditions as diabetes, a foot infection, poor circulation, an unsteady hand or poor vision.

Quick Help for Hurtful Corns. Barry H. Block, D.P.M., of New York City suggests this four-step plan for corn removal:

1. Soak your feet for ten minutes in one-half gallon of warm water into which two tablespoons of household detergent have been added.
2. Dry your foot and rub a few drops of cooking oil into the corn to further soften it.
3. Use a pumice stone, sandpaper or a callus file to gently remove the thickened skin. Use a back and forth sawing motion. Stop at the point where the skin begins to look normal.
4. Cover the corn with a one-eighth inch *non-medicated* felt pad positioned so that the *hole* in the center of the pad is directly over the corn.

Dr. Block cautions against careless do-it-yourself cutting of corns. "Many infections and even loss of toes have resulted from this type of 'bathroom' surgery. Conservative treatment is best left to a podiatrist who has both the experience and the sterile instruments to safely and effectively remove a corn."[57]

Be Cautious of Corn Pads. They can do more harm than good, warns Elizabeth H. Roberts, D.P.M., a podiatrist of New York City. "Don't use those over-the-counter 'corn cures.' They don't cure. They generally contain an acid which destroys the surrounding healthy tissue and often causes an ulceration at the site of the corn. Incidentally, a corn has **no** root, although some 'corn cures' claim to 'remove the root.' There may be a deeper friction at the site of the greatest degree of friction and pressure, but there is **no** root."

Dr. Roberts adds, "If your corn is so painful that you want to protect it until you have the proper treatment, don't buy a corn pad with an oval opening or with an oval depression, which frequently contains an acid preparation. (Remember that the acid is dangerous for tissue.) The oval will cause pressure on the surrounding area, making the corn bulge into the opening."

She suggests, "A much better type of pad to protect a corn is a 'spot' type band-aid, which also has the advantage of a sterile gauze center. Put the sterile gauze directly over the corn. Avoid the rectangular type of band-aid that must be wrapped completely around the toe. The bulk may cause irritation and the constriction may be too great for comfort.[58]

Footwear Can Cause Corns. Protect against corns by wearing properly fitting shoes. **TIPS:** If your feet do not rub against the inside of the shoes, you are not likely to run the risk of corns. **DANGER:** If your shoes are too narrow, you may develop "soft" corns between your toes. These painful lesions are aptly named because they are situated in the moistened interspace of your toes, where they become macerated and soft. *Remedy:* Wear comfortably wide shoes to prevent external pressure from causing the formation of corns.

Soak Away the Pain. Your corn pain may be due to your inflamed or enlarged bursa at the site between the bone and the corn. To ease pain, soak your feet in a solution of comfortably warm water and Epsom salts. This helps bring down the size of the bursa sac and ease some of the pressure on the adjacent sensory nerves. **CAREFUL:** If you put your feet back into tight shoes, the bursa becomes swollen very shortly and you hurt again!

Give Room to Your Toes. Since soft corns are caused by friction of the bones of two adjacent toes, give these toes some room. Separate them. Available are "toe spacers" or "toe separators," which are small pieces of foam you insert between your toes. **CAREFUL:** Do not use cotton between your toes since it will harden and cause more irritation. **TIP:** You could also use good-quality lamb's wool between your toes but not the coarse type that is used in beauty parlors. The better quality is helpful if you draw the strands into a thin, even layer and wrap loosely around one of the toes to provide more room. (Remove the lamb's wool before bathing.)

Better Shoes for Better Foot Health. High-heeled shoes are shaped to fit short and narrow to keep them on, and this can be hurtful to your feet. Wear well-fitting shoes that do not have exceptionally high heels. Midheight heels are more favorable. *Will the Shoe Fit?* Here's a quick test—you want a thumb's-width distance from the end of your longest toe to the end of the shoe. The longest toe is not always the big toe, so do this carefully. You need to have adequate width across the ball of your foot. You should also have sufficient space in your toe box so you feel no pressure across your toes. Shoes should be neither too big nor too small. And . . . always favor natural materials, such as leather, that breathe.

COUGHING

Symptoms

Coughing is a form of vigorous exhalation by which irritant particles in the airways can be expelled. Stimulation of the cough reflexes results in the glottis (space between the two vocal cords) being kept closed until a high expiratory pressure has built up, which is then suddenly released. The medical name is *tussis*. Coughing may be caused by a foreign object lodged somewhere in the lungs or throat, an allergic reaction, a chemical irritant, such as smoke, or a variety of infections that include influenza, sinusitis, pneumonia or a lung disorder. Do not disregard a cough. It is your body's way of disposing of something that does not belong there, whether it is smoke or soap!

You may have a "productive" cough in which waste materials are released so that you have a clearer airway. Leave such coughs alone and help remove wastes by drinking extra liquids.

You may have an "unproductive" cough in which nothing is expelled, and it may keep you awake all night. This may indicate a weakness in your immune system, calling for more liquids and rest. If any cough persists beyond three days, it should be evaluated by your health practitioner. If the cough brings up discolored sputum, medical help is important.

Natural Remedies

If you have a "productive" cough that is dry, take several comfortably warm showers throughout the day to promote a cleansing of waste products. Use a vaporizer to introduce more moisture into your respiratory tract.

Five-Step Coughing-Control Remedy. You can take control of your cough and make it effective, whereby it brings up mucus and helps clear your airways. When you feel a cough coming on, follow these steps:

1. Breathe in deeply.
2. Hold your breath for a second or two.
3. Cough twice, first to loosen the mucus in your airways, then to bring it up.
4. Get rid of mucus. Use strong tissues or paper towels. Swallowing mucus can upset your stomach.

5. Breathe in by sniffing gently.

TIP: The best position for coughing effectively is to sit with your head slightly forward, feet on the floor.

Liquids Soothe Coughing Problems. Lots of liquids will help the waste products become more watery and thus easier to cough up. Plain water is helpful. Warm liquids, too. Plan to quaff at least six glasses of fluid a day to help ease your coughing problem. Avoid caffeine or alcoholic beverages. They function as diuretics and cause loss of fluids . . . when you need to have more!

Licorice Root Tea. Available at health food stores, this tea will soothe irritated throats and ease coughing spasms. It has a natural sedative effect. One or two cups daily will help ease annoying coughs.

Cold-Caused Cough. If your cough is traced to a cold, then you need to ease nasal discomfort. Several squirts of a saline solution up each nostrile can rehydrate the mucous membranes of a "desert nose." There are several ready-to-use preparations available in pharmacies that come in handy squirt bottles. Or, make your own: mix one teaspoon of salt with 2½ cups of warm water. Pour a small amount into your palm and inhale it into your nose. Relief is on the way.

Calm Down that Tickle in Your Throat. It may be tart but it is an effective cough remedy: suck on a whole clove! Within minutes, you will be able to soothe and quiet the irritating tickle that prompts a cough.

Natural Cough Remedy. Gargle with warm salt water. The salt has a modest but beneficial antibacterial benefit, and the feeling is that of soothing relief.

Camphor/Menthol Chest Rub. A gentle rub of this preparation (available in health stores and pharmacies) helps calm a persistent cough. It is welcome at night so you can sleep better. These two ingredients tend to provide soothing comfort and ease the hacking. **CAREFUL:** Never take any chest rub internally. It is exactly what its name says—a chest rub!

Natural Cough Lozenges. If they contain licorice, aromatic oils, such as peppermint or spearmint, or horehound, they dissolve in your throat and help liquefy mucus. They promote breakdown of congestion and wastes. Such lozenges are available in health stores and pharmacies.

Exercise Is Soothing to Your Cough. If you are in otherwise good health, try exercise. It helps loosen up phlegm still stuck in your respiratory tract. The jarring effect of simple exercise such as walking, or moderate calisthenics, will help break up the mucus.

❧

CASE HISTORY—*Coughing Eased with Natural Remedies*

How could Herbert MacD. offer sales presentations when he was constantly interrupting himself with bouts of hacking coughs. Even though he gave up smoking, he still succumbed to coughs after a few sentences of talk. On the phone, he annoyed customers by putting them "on hold" while he broke out into agonizing cough spasms heard all over the office . . . even on the phone lines. Herbert MacD. had mild respiratory problems so could not take medications; neither did he want to further abuse his body with chemicals. How could he conquer the cough that was threatening his livelihood?

An osteopathic physician suggested he "liquefy" his body. He was given a natural prescription: six glasses of plain water daily. No more caffeine beverages; switch to licorice root tea and also peppermint tea. He was told to carry a small pill box with cloves and suck on one when he felt an approaching cough. At night, he used a camphor/menthol chest rub. He boosted his exercise program to 60 minutes nightly. *Results*? Herbert MacD. rebuilt his respiratory tract so that he was no longer susceptible to coughs. The natural remedies had sent the coughs into remission . . . and he was given a promotion because he could now talk sales . . . without interruption. He tripled his quota!

CYSTITIS OR BLADDER DISTRESS

Symptoms

Cystitis is an inflammation of the bladder that has been caused by a urinary tract infection. It is found mostly in women. Its early symptoms are a frequent urge to urinate, a hurtful pain during urination, and the appearance of blood in the urine. The bacteria most often responsible for infection are called *Escherichia coli*—more simply called E. coli. The bacteria usually originates in the bowel, travels across the perineum (the area between the anus and the vagina), and then up the urethra to the bladder.

The bladder has natural defense mechanisms to protect it from infection. Some women are more prone to cystitis, because either their defense mechanisms are inadequate or the bacteria are of a particularly virulent strain that can attach themselves to mucosal surfaces and invade the urinary tract.

More severe attacks are often associated with painful passage of blood in the urine, accompanied by cramp-like pain in the lower abdomen, persisting after the bladder has been emptied.

How Does Bacteria Invade the Bladder? Niels Lauersen, M.D., Professor of Obstetrics and Gynecology at Mt. Sinai Hospital, in New York City, tells us, "Cystitis, a bladder infection, is not technically a sexually transmitted disease, but it can be related to a surge in sexual activity (which is why we have the term 'honeymoon cystitis'). During frequent sexual intercourse, bacteria can be pushed up into a woman's urethra. After the bacteria travel from the urethra into the bladder, a woman feels a pressure to urinate. When she tries to void, she may have either a burning sensation, or blood urine.

"Women who use diaphragms are more commonly afflicted with cystitis because the diaphragm presses against the urethra and distorts the passage. A woman who uses a diaphragm should urinate before and after intercourse to relieve the pressure on her bladder."

Natural Remedies

Dr. Lauersen suggests, "If a woman with cystitis increases her intake of vitamin C and drinks a lot of cranberry juice—both also good for preventing cystitis—she will be making her urine more acidic and hastening her cure."[59]

Why Cranberry Juice Is Helpful. It contains *quinolic acid*, which makes the urine inhospitable to E. coli, the germs that most often infect the bladder.

Drink Lots of Liquids. Plan to have at least six glasses a day, and void frequently. Usually bacteria entering the bladder are flushed out during urination. But if you allow yourself to become dehydrated, the E. coli bacteria get "stuck." They colonize rapidly—doubling every 20 minutes—producing the infection. Drink lots of water daily!

Soapy Bubble Baths Could Be Irritating. Bubble baths and soapy water could cause skin irritations that mimic urinary infections by making voiding uncomfortable. If you notice this, go easy on such products.

Personal Hygiene. Void completely before and after intercourse. While in the bathroom the second time, drink another glass of water. Keep clean! Wipe from front to back after elimination to keep bowel bacteria away from the urethra.

Avoid Alcohol. It is believed that alcohol irritates an infected bladder, so to be on the safe side, skip the drinks!

Finally, women prone to this infection should take special precautions when they are well and sexually active. And if cystitis is diagnosed, it is best to avoid sex.

CASE HISTORY—*"Embarrassed" By Infection—Feels Depressed*

Was her marriage facing a standstill? Linda Y. observed the presence of blood in her urine. There was increasing hurtful pain. Her gynecologist diagnosed cystitis. Linda Y. had to abstain from sex; rightfully so, since women do not contract cystitis from their sexual partners—although intercourse could provoke an infection. She felt embarrassed and also depressed (in her own words), because she felt her marriage could fall apart. She could not take antibiotics because of side effects, such as yeast infections, since drug therapy could eradicate "friendly" vaginal bacteria that keep yeast (a fungus) from growing. She was prone to yeast infections. What to do?

Linda Y.'s gynecologist asked her to follow the increased water program. She also was careful to be very clean. She then took recommended vitamin C on a daily basis along with several glasses of cranberry juice. It took four weeks until her symptoms eased . . . and in six weeks, she went on a "second honeymoon," because these natural remedies—amazingly simple—were equally as amazingly effective. She was healed! Life became romantic again!

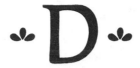

DEPRESSION

Symptoms

Warning signs are general sadness, difficulty in making decisions, an inability to concentrate; reading and writing become difficult. Low self-esteem; unable to make yourself feel better regardless of what you do. A feeling of hopelessness, that nothing will improve the situation. Changes in eating, sleeping and sexual habits. Lethargy and slowness of speech. Depressed people tend to withdraw from others, not because they want to be alone, but because they are afraid to be among others. They are overly sensitive to words and actions of others. Excessive crying, restlessness, irritability or overactivity, low energy or slowed thinking, and thoughts of suicide or death.

Some depression is common in all our lives. It is usually caused by a life crisis, such as the loss of someone we are close to, moving away from close friends, the break-up of a marriage, and so on. Almost any major change in our lives creates stress. It is when the stress-caused depression hangs on for a long time, and we become increasingly unable to function in our normal roles, that the ailment is serious, requiring help.

Natural Remedies

If you're feeling melancholy, down in the dumps, some basic techniques can help brighten up your feeling of the blues. Remake your lifestyle with these basic depression-easing remedies:

Keep Yourself Active. Erwin DiCyan, Ph.D., noted psychotherapist of Brooklyn, New York, urges that you "do something to stimulate yourself. Hanging around the house and feeling sorry for yourself will make you more depressed. Get *away* from your home. No matter what you do, as long as it is *active*. Try taking a walk, a bicycle ride. Visit a friend. Play a game of cards, checkers, or anything you like. Do **NOT** look at television because that is not being active."

What Fun Things Do You Like to Do? Dr. DiCyan explains, "I tell my patients to write down a list of things they enjoy. Of course, to a depressed person, nothing looks enjoyable. So I suggest writing down activities that used to be enjoyable. Then I advise: pick one—and do it! Getting involved in physical activities, if they are fun, is a great way to get out of the blues."

Talk It Out. Relieve the pressures of depression by airing your feelings. "Share your feelings with someone who cares and is sympathetic," suggests the psychotherapist. "Tell what is on your mind. The mere act of talking it out is helpful."

Put Big Decisions on "Hold." Dr. DiCyan says, "You should not trust your judgment if depressed. Put off any major decisions until you're feeling better; otherwise, you are likely to make the *wrong* decision and that will depress you further."

Avoid Conflict with Others. Being depressed, you have a tendency to snap at others. Doing so means others will snap back at you. "Try to keep away from conflicts. Avoid crowds because a wrong word or move and you could fly off the handle," cautions Dr. DiCyan. "Disputes and debates are best to be avoided."

Keep Away from Food. An eating binge might make you feel good "but it also adds inches to your waistline and if you become overweight, you have less self-esteem and more problems," cautions Dr. DiCyan. "Keep yourself active so you have less of an urge to eat. More physical activity helps chase away the blues and also control your appetite."[60]

Nutritional Program Brightens Your Mood. With a simple nutritional formula, you may help brighten your mood. Priscilla Slagle, M.D., Associate Clinical Professor at the University of California, Los Angeles, emphasizes the use of several nutrients to help you overcome depression. She recommends:

Take 1,000 to 3,000 milligrams of L-tyrosine (amino acid) first thing in the morning (on an empty stomach).

Take a B-complex vitamin supplement 30 minutes later with your breakfast.

Benefit: Dr. Slagle explains that L-tyrosine changes in the brain to norepinephrine, a natural substance that gives you a happier mood, better self-esteem and ambition. The B-complex vitamins, especially vitamin B_6, helps your body metabolize the amino acids.

"I don't know anyone with a mild problem who has not responded to the treatment," says Dr. Slagle. It is important for you to seek medical approval, however, before starting supplement therapy.[61]

Food for Your "Depressed" Brain. If your brain is deficient in

neurotransmitters (chemical messengers) such as norepinephrine or serotonin, you may have feelings of depression. Most drugs used by psychia-
trists to treat depression are aimed at increasing levels of one or both
of these brain chemical messengers. You may also raise brain levels of
norepinephrine and serotonin with the use of the amino acids of phenylalanine and tryptophan. Both raise brain levels of the messengers so that
you have relief from the symptoms of depression and mood swings. Both
of these amino acids are found in protein foods and are also available
as supplements, to be used with the approval of your health practitioner.

Niacin Helps Improve Your Mood. This B-complex vitamin helps
produce energy metabolism and is involved in stimulating the manufacture of brain chemicals. Many patients diagnosed with mental unrest
are found to be deficient in niacin. This vitamin spares the tryptophan
in the brain for more serotonin production and helps ease feelings of
depression. When niacin is included in a B-complex supplement, it helps
establish the equilibrium needed for correcting symptoms of depression.

CASE HISTORY—*Nutritional Therapy Rescues Victim of Depression
from Hospital Confinement*

Victor F. could not shake off his persistent sad or "empty" feelings. He
was pessimistic, troubled with sleep disturbances, expressed feelings of
hopelessness. He had difficulty in concentrating, remembering and making decisions. He was alienated from his family; at times, Victor F. felt
that if he took his own life, he would be "doing them a favor." When
he had these symptoms for over two weeks, he was classified as depressed.
His family was worried he might take his own life and considered putting
him under hospital supervision. They could not risk leaving him out of
sight. But Victor F. developed so many side effects from prescribed medications, he could not undergo prolonged treatment of this sort. A relative
had almost succumbed to depression until he was treated by an orthomolecular psychiatrist who specialized in correcting the disorder with emphasis on nutrition. Here was a ray of hope.

The psychiatrist diagnosed Victor F. as being nutritionally deficient
in the amino acids of phenylalanine, tyrosine and tryptophan. He needed
to have his niacin levels improved, too. With the use of nutritional therapy
with emphasis on these elements, his brain levels of norepinephrine
and serotonin were raised so that he became more optimistic. In nine
weeks, he felt more hopeful, could sleep better, had sharper powers of
thought, and felt warm love toward his family. He would no longer even
think of suicide and felt embarrassed if it was even mentioned. By the

end of eleven weeks, Victor F. was healed of his depression, thanks to nutritional programs, and was ready to restructure his life to face a brand new future! He had been "saved" from hospital confinement with this orthomolecular approach using nutrition and improved lifestyles.

DERMATITIS

Symptoms

Itch . . . scratch . . . scratch. In brief, this is dermatitis (also known as eczema), a general term for inflammation of the skin. It consists of a diffuse rash with itching. Symptoms include rash, itching, burning, dryness, blemishes. Dermatitis is caused by chafing of the skin by external irritants such as gasoline, turpentine or fertilizers; excessive exposure to sunlight; detergents, soaps, or other chemicals that dry or degrease the skin; cement, various plants, insects or industrial chemicals. Dermatitis may be traced to allergies, nervousness, or prolonged use of medications.

Natural Remedies

Your skin reacts if you are nutritionally deficient because cell turnover time is short. Skin cells are produced, die and are replaced by new cells within a few days. The short lifespan of these cells is a reflection of the importance of nutrition. Some important skin-healing nutrients that may cure dermatitis include:

Vitamin A. Needed to protect against dry, scaly and rough skin common in dermatitis. Include vitamin A foods in small amounts to help correct any possible deficiency. These include carrots, cantaloupe, peaches, squash, tomatoes, all green and yellow fruits, vegetables, dairy products.

Vitamin D. Helps relieve scaling skin and creates smoothness and relief from itching. Food sources include seafood, fish liver oil, egg yolk (high in cholesterol!). If you take supplements, do not exceed the RDA 400 international units, unless supervised by your health practitioner.

Vitamin B Complex. This family of vitamins will help heal dermatitis-like symptoms such as soreness and burning of the skin, scaly or darkened patches, itching, numbness or tingling of the skin. Food sources include brewer's yeast, whole grains, legumes, wheat germ, whole brown rice, soybeans, organ meats (high in cholesterol).

Vitamin C. Needed for the formation and maintenance of collagen, the connective tissue that holds cells together. Helps protect against dry or scaly skin or poor wound healing. Food sources include fresh fruits (especially citrus), vegetables, green and red peppers.

Zinc. An oft-neglected mineral that is needed for the absorption of an essential nutrient—linoleic acid, the fatty acid that improves your skin. Food sources include brewer's yeast, beans, nuts, seeds, wheat germ, seafood.

Linoleic Acid. Most helpful in healing blotchy areas, especially those near the oil-secreting glands, folds of the nose, lips, forehead, cheeks. Food sources include nuts, wheat germ, vegetable oils.

To help you improve your resistance to dermatitis, here are helpful remedies offered by Jerome Z. Litt, M.D., of Case Western Reserve University of Medicine, in Cleveland, Ohio:

- Never use soap! It removes the natural oils from your already overdry skin. Use a soapless cleanser, or a soap substitute.
- Take baths and showers in lukewarm—not hot—water; add soothing bath oils to the water for excessively dry, scaly skin. And when you dry, dry by patting—not by rubbing.
- Keep your fingernails short and clean.
- Avoid sudden extremes of temperature and any violent exercise that causes sweating. Going from a hot to a cold or from a cold to a hot environment will trigger the itching response.
- Keep your relative humidity above 40 percent—winter and summer—to protect an already dry skin from becoming completely dehydrated.
- Eliminate fuzzy, rough and woolen clothing because they worsen dermatitis. Use soft, loose, cotton clothing.
- Dispose of furry and fuzzy toys, and feather pillows.
- While it may seem cruel, removing household pets, particularly longhaired dogs and cats, is a must.
- Don't work around or expose yourself to dust, industrial chemicals, fumes, sprays, cutting oils, paints, varnishes and solvents. All of these will worsen your dermatitis.
- Avoid all cosmetics, cleansers, body oils and lotions that contain

lanolin. Lanolin is good for sheep but bad for humans. It causes allergies, plugs up oil glands (causing acne) and aggravates dermatitis. (Besides, why use a product on your skin that is advertised as great for polishing shoes and cleaning pots?)

- Avoid colds and other respiratory infections. They lower the resistance of your skin and make your dermatitis worse.

- Don't wear rubber gloves for household chores. Even the cotton-lined varieties "sweat" when immersed in hot water, thereby leaching out the chemicals and stabilizers in the rubber, which only exacerbate the eczema on the fingers. If you find that you must do the housework and dishes with rubber gloves, get cotton liners and wear them at all times under the cotton-lined rubber gloves.

- Avoid exposing yourself to people who have cold sores (fever blisters). The virus that causes cold sores can cause serious eruptions in those who have dermatitis.

- Avoid over-the-counter salves and lotions containing benzocaine and antihistamines.

- Do not use petroleum jelly and other greasy ointments. They tend to intensify the itching by preventing the evaporation of sweat.

- Whenever possible, avoid emotional stress and tension. You may find that a flare-up of your condition was actually triggered by some conflict, anxiety or stressful situation. There is no other skin condition where "nerves" play a greater role.

- Try not to scratch. Not only will scratching aggravate your condition, but it can break and damage your skin, thus contributing to secondary bacterial infection.

"Above all," advises Dr. Litt, "try to be patient and keep a positive attitude. Despite the agony it can cause, dermatitis is not a serious disorder. If you can learn to live with it and keep the rash under control, chances are it will fade itself out as it goes into remission. If, however, your rash persists, and the itching is uncontrollable, see your dermatologist."[62]

Soak in Oatmeal. Soothe your itching inflammation with a soak in an oatmeal bath. Here's how: add two cups of colloidal oatmeal (available at health food stores and most pharmacies) into a tub of lukewarm water. Enjoy a soak for about 20 minutes. You'll emerge feeling much better. *NOTE*: The term *colloidal* means the oatmeal has been ground into a fine powder that remains suspended in water.

Cool Off Dermatitis with Oatmeal Soap. Since you have overly dry skin, you want to keep clean and avoid oil loss, yet you should not use commercial soap. Try Oatmeal Soap as a substitute. Wrap colloidal oatmeal in a clean handkerchief. Tighten an elastic band around the top. Dunk it in lukewarm water. Wring it out. Use it as you would an ordinary washcloth. Gently rub as if a soap. You'll clean your skin and preserve the needed oil at the same time. It's Oatmeal Soap!

Cold Milk Compress. Soothe itching with this compress. In a glass of milk, add several ice cubes and let stand five minutes. Then dip a thin piece of cotton or a gauze pad in the milk. Apply to the irritated skin for three minutes. Resoak the cloth and reapply; continue this Cold Milk Process for 15 minutes. It should soothe the agonizing itch before the end of the day. Otherwise, see your dermatologist.

DIARRHEA

Symptoms

A condition in which waste matter is discharged from the bowel more often than usual and in a more or less liquid state. Diarrhea results when one of a number of viruses infect the bowel, making it weep fluid. There may be accompanying cramping abdominal pain. Mild forms are common and insignificant, apart from perhaps one day away from work and a few minor discomforts. If it lasts for weeks or months, then it can be an indication of major illness. The more serious form of diarrhea may be accompanied by blood, slime, or undigested food in the wastes.

Natural Remedies

In most situations, the best remedy is to do nothing, but stop eating and drink a great deal to replace lost fluid.

Hold Back Milk Products. Insufficiency of the enzyme lactase which digests milk sugar, is a common but frequently overlooked cause of diarrhea. If you have repeated, unexplained bouts of diarrhea, you might stop consuming milk products for one week, or two, to see if the condition clears up. **TIP:** Lactase deficiency may be overcome if you pretreat milk with the enzyme just before consuming milk products. Milk-digesting lactase tablets are available at most health stores.

Sorbitol May Be to Blame. This synethetic sweetener is found in many diet products (ice cream, soft drinks, pastries, etc.) and, if ingested in large amounts, could cause diarrhea. Symptoms vary from one person to the next. *Problem*: Sorbitol is not absorbed by the small intestine; it reaches the large intestine intact. This reaction draws fluid into the large intestine to cause diarrhea. *Solution*: Avoid any products which list sorbitol as an ingredient!

Drink More Liquids. Replenish lost water by drinking lots of liquids. Time-honored chicken soup is good because it has natural sodium which is easily absorbed to make up for your loss. Carbonated beverages and plain crackers also help replace lost electrolytes needed for balancing your body chemistry.

Tea Tames Diarrhea. Ordinary tea may help tame your diarrhea. It has tannic acid, an astringent, believed to protect the intestinal membranes from irritating substances.

Fiber Is Helpful. Fiber-containing foods can be an effective natural remedy for diarrhea (and for constipation) because it normalizes intestinal transit time.

The most immediate risk associated with diarrhea is that of dehydration, therefore it is essential to consume as much liquid as is comfortably tolerated. Ordinarily you would want to avoid salt and sugar, but in this condition, a temporary adjustment would be helpful. You could try the following natural remedies:

Rehydration Beverage. Add one teaspoon of sugar and a pinch of salt to one quart of room temperature water. Stir and drink throughout the day.

Liquid Replacement Drink. Add one-half teaspoon of honey and a pinch of table salt to eight ounces of natural fruit juice. Stir well and drink slowly.

Both of these beverages contain sufficient amounts of glucose and electrolytes to replace those lost by your body.

Antibiotics, Diarrhea, Yogurt. Wide-spectrum or multiple antibiotics can cause stubborn diarrhea because the drugs wipe out beneficial intestinal bacteria. To counteract their effect, live-culture yogurt and acidophilus milk (both with *lactobacillus bacteria*) are helpful. Yogurt positively influences the ratio of good to bad bacteria in your intestines. Yogurt also disposes of the *clostridium* bugs—the culprit behind antibiotic-induced diarrhea. Make yogurt part of your diarrhea-healing program.

Bananas Are Helpful. Bananas help fight certain types of diarrhea. They perform a two-pronged effect: they restore lost potassium and add fiber, which absorbs water in the stool. Furthermore, the fiber adds bulk and stabilizes the region.

Hints, Tips, Suggestions. AVOID carbonated beverages because they accelerate the contractions of intestinal muscles, pushing food down into the gastrointestinal tract all the more swiftly. Avoid coffee (regular or decaffeinated) because it acts as natural diuretic. Apples and bananas contain pectin, which help make the stool firmer and recovery all the better. As you begin to feel better, slowly introduce applesauce, bananas, then toast and bland foods.

DIGESTIVE UPSET

Symptoms

Poor appetite, nausea, feeling of fullness or stomach ache, diarrhea and, perhaps, fever. *Important* warning signs include: stomach pains that are severe, last a long time, are recurring, or come with shaking, chills and cold, clammy skin. Be alert to recurrent nausea, a sudden change in bowel habits, pain or difficulty in swallowing food, continuing loss of appetite, or unexpected weight loss.

Digestion and the Older Person. The diet of older folks is often less than optimal. The aging process tends to lessen the sensitivity of taste buds; older people tend to eat less because food does not taste as good as it used to. There may be problems chewing because of tooth loss or ill-fitting dentures. Physical disabilities may make shopping and food preparation too difficult. Medications may also lessen appetite. And . . . many older people get too little exercise, especially when there is a physical condition that makes exercising difficult. All these factors contribute to a malfunctioning of the digestive system.

Natural Remedies

A basic program calls for these steps:

1. Drink eight or more glasses of water a day. Besides the other bodily functions that require it, water plays an essential role in digestion. Adequate water is especially important with a high-fiber diet.
2. Daily exercise is needed. You will be able to promote fitness of your digestive problems with at least 60 minutes of exercise daily.

3. Your food program should include proper amounts of fruits, vegetables, and whole grains. Boost your intake of dietary fiber from a good selection of fresh foods as well as whole grains, fruits and vegetables, and legumes.

4. Be alert to causes of digestive upset. Avoid smoking—the tar and smoke irritants stimulate secretion of saliva as they are inhaled into the body, and this irritates the stomach lining, causing upset. Some prescription and non-prescription drugs may irritate your stomach lining and should be discussed with your physician. Strain from stress and nervousness prompts the stomach to secrete excessive amounts of digestive juices (acid). If there is no food available for these juices to break down, they irritate your stomach lining. If you are under constant strain with frequently recurring upset stomach, you are releasing too much acid, which can literally eat away a part of the stomach lining, causing a gastric ulcer.

How to Ease Digestive Upset. If you have a mild upset, refrain from eating for several hours and the symptoms should go away. To protect against upset, eat slowly and chew your food thoroughly so your stomach has a chance to work normally. Do not overload your stomach. Stay away from spicy or difficult-to-digest foods.

Be Careful of Alcohol. It has an irritating effect that can cause inflammation of the mucous membrane surface of the stomach lining. This brings on a feeling of digestive upset and nausea. **DANGER:** Because alcohol stimulates secretion of gastric acid and can also act to delay the process that allows the acid to leave the stomach, a backup of acid often results. Over a long period of time, this excess acid irritates and damages the stomach lining.

Herbs Help Heal Hurtful Digestive System. Most natural flavoring and seasoning herbs promote a flow of digestive juices in the stomach and intestine, thereby boosting the efficiency with which fats are broken down into fatty acids and nutrients are absorbed by your body. Certain herb partnerships reflect this soothing reaction:

- Rosemary helps the digestion of fatty lamb.
- Fennel assists the digestion of oily fish.
- Horseradish improves the digestion of beef.

Natural Digestive Tonics. Add one tablespoon of ground aniseed to one cup of milk. Drink this twice a day to help improve your digestive system. Hot peppermint tea after a meal is very soothing to your process of digestion.

If you must eat rich foods, finish with a dish of digestive herbs including aniseed, caraway, dill and fennel seeds for better digestion. Try to avoid heavy meals, though.

Relax and Have Healthier Digestion. Unwind . . . ease away from stress . . . remain calm, and your digestive system will serve you all the better. Whether you use meditation, self-hypnosis, or visualization, if it helps you gain control over your emotions, use it! Your digestive system is a built-in barometer that reacts to stress and strain. If you cannot calm yourself before eating . . . don't eat until you can calm yourself! Otherwise, your digestive system pays the penalty!

DIVERTICULAR DISORDERS

Symptoms

You are over 40 and have been bothered for some time with abdominal cramps, gas and diarrhea alternating with constipation. You are diagnosed as having a diverticular disorder. It is an acquired problem, traced to processed foods that are low in fiber, needed to ease colon tension and help it expand when eliminating waste.

The name comes from the Latin word *diverticulum* which means a "small diversion from the normal path." With a diverticular disorder, balloon-like sacs or tiny, grapelike pouches called *diverticula* develop in the walls of the colon (large intestine). These tiny pouches are formed when pressure causes the inside wall of the colon to bulge out through the weak spots in the outer wall. This might be compared to a bicycle inner tube, which bulges out through a defect in the tire.

Diverticulosis is a disorder in which these pouches are present. Tiny pockets of the membrane lining of the colon are pushed out from the inside of the intestinal wall to form the small sacs. Often there are no symptoms, and you may be unaware that you have it.

Diverticulitis is a serious disorder in which some of these pouches have become irritated or infected, also inflamed. The symptoms may be pain or even bleeding. There could be changes in bowel habits. If not treated, it can become very serious. The inflammation can cause swelling and ultimately obstruct the colon.

Natural Remedies

Diverticular disorders are traced to the low fiber intake of our modern times. Food is highly refined, over-processed, and lacking in natural fiber. A deficiency of fiber leads to constipation, with small hard stools that do not fill out the colon. The colon then develops areas of spasms which force the pouches through the muscle wall.

A high-fiber program will not only prevent the development of diverticular disorders but will correct it promptly once it is established. This same high-fiber program helps prevent and correct constipation caused by improper diet. To boost fiber intake:

1. Eat more bran via whole grains, cereals, muffins, brown rice, breads.

2. Increase intake of raw fruit (including skin and pulp), with emphasis upon apples, grapes, melons, nectarines, oranges, peaches, pears, plums, figs.

3. If you eat cooked or dried fruit, try applesauce, apricots, prunes, raisins.

4. Boost intake of raw vegetables such as broccoli, cabbage, carrots, cauliflower, celery, lettuce.

5. Enjoy cooked, high-fiber vegetables, such as asparagus, broccoli, Brussels sprouts, cauliflower, corn, potatoes, squash, string beans, turnips.

Bran Protects Against Diverticular Disorders. You may start eating two or three tablespoons of bran cereal in the morning and gradually build up to one-half cup a day. This is often more comfortable on a slower basis, because you may not tolerate high-fiber foods very well. *Note:* Bran is the outer coating of whole wheat grain, which is removed in the processing of grain. Emphasize daily intake of bran via whole grain foods to help control your condition.

Peas and Beans Are Good Source of Fiber. Include peas, beans, and lentils in your fiber-boosting program. Other tasty sources include baked potatoes, cooked broccoli tops, raw mushrooms, whole wheat pasta, and popcorn.

The benefit of fiber is that it draws water into the stool so the movements are smoother. You can "sneak" more fiber into meals without really noticing with these nutritional remedies:

• Eat whole grain breads and cereals instead of those that are refined or processed.

• Boost the use of fruit for desserts.

- Baked fruits (peaches, pears, apples) should have the skins intact.
- Switch to using any kind of beans instead of beef in casseroles, stews or chili.
- Barley and brown rice should be part of most vegetable soups.
- More liquids should be taken with your fiber-boosting plan. Drinking at least six glasses of water is helpful in moisturizing the fiber and overcoming constipation, which is frequently associated with diverticular disorders.
- CAREFUL: Avoid foods with small seeds or sharp particles (such as nuts) if you have this disorder. They may lodge in the pouches and cause distress.

Daily Exercise Is A Must. If you are sedentary, you may have flabby intestinal muscles and a slowing of the propulsion effect. Tone up your entire body. Try aerobics, calisthenics, walking up a few flights of stairs daily. A brisk 60-minute walk is a great (and easy) way to exercise your sluggish colon. Do it daily!

❧

CASE HISTORY—*Corrects Painful Colon Upset with Natural Remedies*

When she became sales supervisor, Leona Z. had less and less time to go to the bathroom when necessary. She ate "fast foods" and let herself become fiber-deficient. When she had problems with constipation, she tried laxatives. She developed bouts of colitis, which worsened with more laxatives. When she experienced pain, she sought help from a gastroenterologist. He advised her to establish regularity under all circumstances. "Your health comes before your job!" Then he put her on a high-fiber diet which included whole grain foods and much more of such meatless sources as beans, peas, whole-grain pasta, raw fruits and vegetables.

Boosting her fiber intake and establishing regularity helped Leona Z. soothe her diverticular distress in a short while. She soon was free of pain, cramps and colitis on this simple but natural program. She was later diagnosed as being "saved from surgery," since her pouches were almost eroding into blood vessels to cause perforation and bleeding. Leona Z. felt "young again" as she continued her career . . . but thereafter her health was always given priority!

DUST, ALLERGIES TO

Symptoms

House dust—a nuisance to the conscientious housekeeper—is also the source of misery for allergic persons who are bothered by sneezing, a runny nose, wheezing and shortness of breath, watery, itching eyes. This condition is often called allergic rhinitis.

House Dust Mite: Invisible Invader. Actually, the allergy is not to dust itself but to a microscopic, eight-legged creature called the house dust mite. You are not allergic to the mite itself but to the tiny, tough pellets of waste matter it excretes after dining on flakes of skin from people or pets. House dust mites are found in almost every kind of natural and synthetic fiber. Their favorite places are mattresses, armchairs, couches, carpets, pillows and even stuffed toys.

Dust mites thrive when the temperature and humidity are in the 70's. If you conserve energy by sealing leaks in your homes, adding carpets and drapes for insulation, you favor the survival and reproduction of dust mites. Although the dust mite lives only two to four months, during that time it produces about 200 times its own body weight in waste. Over time, the waste breaks down to tiny particles, mixes in with dust, and is then inhaled.

Unfortunately, vacuuming does not solve the problem—90 percent of house dust mites remain in upholstery, mattresses, and carpets even after a thorough vacuuming. Therefore, to stop allergic reactions from occurring, house dust mites and their waste need to be eliminated from the home.

Natural Remedies

Allergy specialists with the Baylor College of Medicine, in Houston, Texas, offer these suggestions to protect against dust attacks:

In the home, start with your bedroom: it is the single most-important room in the allergy sufferer's life. Beds are havens for house dust and mold. If you awake most mornings sneezing or stuffed up, it's probably your bed. Change the bedding often. Clean your mattress by hard suction vacuuming. Vacuum under the bed at least twice a month. Vacuum your whole house regularly in order to keep the amount of dust low. The heater and air conditioner filters should be cleaned at least once a month when in use, more often with heavier use.

All houses have some mold, too. This can be controlled somewhat by regular cleaning and vacuuming. Mold is a powerful allergen, and is most bothersome in humid areas.

Beware of Mold Sources: Mattresses, feather and foam pillows, books, cardboard boxes, shoes, houseplants, bathroom cabinets, shower curtains, storage closets, paper products and wall paper, garbage containers. *Remedy*: A disinfectant spray or plain rubbing alcohol can be used to wipe away and kill mold.

Certain foods that contain mold—beer, red wine, aged cheese, canned tomatoes, and mushrooms—should probably be avoided by the mold-sensitive person.[63]

How to Help Dust-Proof Your House. Breathe easier with these suggestions from various specialists:

- Enclose your mattress in heavy vinyl plastic; cover with a washable mattress pad. Keep away from fuzzy or electric blankets.
- Every 10 days, wash bedding in water heated to at least 130°F. (Mites survive washing in cooler water.)
- Pillows should be made of polyester fiberfill. Best to avoid feather or kapok.
- Clear away all "dust catchers" where you spend most of your time— and that includes the bedroom.
- If you have to do your own cleaning, wear a mask to protect against inhaling dust. And, when finished, go outside for about 30 minutes so the airborne dust can settle.
- Every month, clean your heating and/or air-conditioning filters.
- Best floors are made of wood or vinyl. Cover only with washable area rugs. If carpeting has to be used, plan to vacuum regularly. (It does not get rid of live mites, but helps remove surface dust.)
- Clean floors, woodwork and furniture with dust-removing polish.
- Avoid collecting stuffed animals, unnecessary pillows, books, magazines, and knick-knacks. They attract dust . . . so does upholstery.
- In humid weather, run an air-conditioner or dehumidifier. This is especially important from spring through fall when mites proliferate more than any other time of the year.
- Considering a move? If possible, select a residence with wood or vinyl. **TIP:** Try to avoid basement living areas or ground-floor bedrooms, which are built over cement and very damp.
- In warm weather, keep room temperatures below 70°F and relative humidity below 50 percent by using an air-conditioner and, if neces-

sary, a dehumidifier. Mites die when the relative humidity drops to 40 to 50 percent.

- Walls should be painted or covered with washable wallpaper. Closet doors should be kept closed.

- In addition to carrying out a dust avoidance program, try to avoid contact with such inhalants as insect sprays, fresh paint, tobacco smoke, and fresh tar. These substances have irritating effects on already inflamed membranes. High concentrations of air pollutants can also cause discomfort in those with dust allergy.

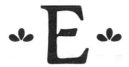

EARS

Symptoms

It can steal up on you so imperceptibly that at first you are completely unaware of it; otherwise, it can strike suddenly and condemn you to a lifetime of silence. Hearing impairment! Typical symptoms include earache, ringing in the ears, difficulty in hearing certain sounds, abnormal ear noises, dizziness, discomfort or pain in the ears and/or head.

Natural Remedies

Here are some common and uncommon hearing problems and helpful natural remedies.

Wax in Ear. A natural secretion that has a protective function. Some people's glands secrete excessive wax. When wax accumulates, it can block the ear canal completely, causing temporary hearing loss. *Remedy*: Small amounts of soft wax can be removed by gently using a moistened swab at the opening of the ear canal. Large amounts or hardened wax should be removed by a health practitioner.

Otitis Media. The medical name of bacterial or viral infections in the middle ear. The chief symptom is an earache. Fever may accompany the problem. *Remedy*: Boost the intake of nutrients, such as vitamins A, B complex and C, and minerals, such as potassium and magnesium, to help overcome the infection. Warm beverages help clear up any congestion to facilitate healing.

Tinnitus. A ringing sound in the ears, although there may be hissing, buzzing or roaring. The mildest causes are traced to wax buildup against the eardrum. *Remedy*: A home remedy is to use a few drops of vegetable oil to soften the earwax and wash it out. The liquid left inside will bubble away at the wax and soften it for removal. Next, fill a rubber bulb syringe with body temperature water. Hold your head over a bowl, squirt the water *gently* into your ear canal. *No pressure!* Easy does it. Turn your head to one side and the water with the wax will wash out. Let your ear dry at room temperature. No rubbing after this remedy.

Meniere's Disease. Caused by an abnormal pressure in the fluid of the inner ear, which in turn disturbs the organ of equilibrium, which is situated in your inner ear. Symptoms include dizziness, nausea and loss of hearing accompanied by ringing in the ears. *Remedy*: Avoid salt which tends to absorb water and cause distress. You may also be sensitive to salt. Reduce stress, which could bring on attacks of vertigo or dizziness. Relaxation exercises and a lifestyle change is often most helpful.

Dizziness. You feel lightheaded, unsteady or giddy; this could be traced to an inner ear problem or vertigo. *Remedy*: A set of remedies is offered by the American Academy of Otolaryngology:

1. Avoid rapid changes in position, especially from lying down to standing up or turning around from one side to the other.
2. Avoid extremes of head motion (especially looking up) or rapid head motion (especially turning or twisting).
3. Eliminate or decrease use of products that impair circulation, e.g., nicotine, caffeine, and salt.
4. Minimize your exposure to circumstances that precipitate your dizziness, such as stress and anxiety, or substances to which you are allergic.
5. Avoid hazardous activities when you are dizzy, such as driving an automobile or operating dangerous equipment, or climbing a step ladder.[64]

Noise: Danger to Hearing. It's everywhere, disturbing your peace, jarring your nerves, damaging your hearing. The louder the noise, the more dangerous it is to hearing health. Noise is hurtful and can lead to permanent hearing impairment and loss. Turn down the volume. Keep away from noisy areas, if at all possible. Wearing earplugs is a good way to preserve your hearing. Keep away from motorized tools, loud music and noisy regions. Remember: if you cannot carry on a conversation in the presence of any type of noise, it is too loud for your ears and can potentially cause hearing loss.

EMPHYSEMA

Symptoms

In this condition, there is trapped air in the tissues. In pulmonary emphysema the air sacs (alveoli) of the lungs are enlarged and damaged, which reduces the surface area for the exchange of oxygen and carbon dioxide. Severe emphysema causes breathlessness, which is made worse by infection. This ailment is known to be particularly common in men and is associated with chronic bronchitis, smoking, and advancing age. It is also known as "chronic obstructive lung disease" or COLD. The major symptom is that of "air hunger"—the hard work of breathing requiring all available muscles accompanying each breath, especially when exhaling. Air gets trapped in the lungs, causing hyperventilation, often resulting in a "barrel-shaped" chest.

Natural Remedies

Air pollution and smoking are two of the major causes of emphysema, and should be avoided. Inhaled pollutants increase formation of toxic chemicals in the body that destroy elastin, a key component that gives resiliency to lung tissue. You could also be harmed by sidestream smoke of other smokers, so keep away from such dangers.

Keep Yourself Active. Walking is a great total body exercise. Tone up the muscles in your upper extremities by using one-pound or two-pound handweights and move the muscles of your neck, upper shoulders and chest. This is important to help keep these muscles more vigorous to meet the challenges of daily activities.

Simple Breathing Remedies. Try pursed-lip breathing, swimming in moderate temperatures. Balloon inflation games, blowing ping pong balls, will help improve the capacity of your lungs. You will improve muscle tone and slow progression of COLD.

Smaller Meals Are Soothing. With more serious emphysema, there is more blockage of the airflow as the lungs expand with trapped air. These enlarged lungs press into your stomach, restricting expansion of your stomach. Therefore, you will be easing distress by eating several smaller meals throughout the day. Aim for six small ones, rather than three large ones. CAREFUL: In this situation, prolonged digestion dispatches oxygen and blood to your stomach, pulling them away from other body parts where they are needed. *Remember*: protect against airflow blockage with several smaller meals throughout the day.

Control Your Weight. Get rid of the excess pounds, which tend to retain fluid. More energy is used to carry excess weight, and you'll feel drained. Select low-fat and high-protein foods to trim your waistline so you'll breathe better.

Breathe in Rhythm. Take a moment to check your breathing rhythm. Chaotic? Short bursts with large bursts? Gasps and groans? Normalize your breathing in a rhythmic pattern so your lungs are able to provide comfort to your respiratory tract.

Breathe from Your Stomach. It's efficient and soothing. Babies do it by instinct; see how their bellies rise and fall with each breath? *How To Do It*: Lie down on your back. Have someone put a reasonably heavy telephone book on your belly. Breathe. See if your book-covered belly goes up and down. If not, make corrections!

Clean Your "Dirty" Lungs. Set aside 30 minutes each day for this lung-washing exercise. Pucker your lips. Blow out slowly. Try to breathe out *twice as long* as it took you to breathe in. ***Benefit:*** You will help clean the stale-dirty air from your lungs, allowing fresh air to enter.

Nutritional Remedies. Smoking and pollution destroy certain vitamins. Oxidants penetrate through your lungs to destroy cells. You need anti-oxidant vitamins such as vitamins A, C, E, and the minerals of selenium and zinc. Be sure to get your vitamin RDA . . . and discuss additional potencies with your health practitioner.

Don't Overdo It. You surely should keep active, but know your limitations. Go about your tasks quietly and calmly. Rearrange your work area for more efficiency. You'll be rewarded with more energy . . . and breath, too!

If You Must Lift. Exhale through pursed lips when you lift. Inhale while you rest. Going upstairs or otherwise climbing? Exhale through pursed lips as you go up . . . inhale as you rest.

Loosen Up. Your clothing, that is. Allow your chest and abdomen to expand freely. No tight belts, bras, girdles. Men might prefer suspenders instead of tight belts. Women may find camisoles more comfortable than bras.

ENDOMETRIOSIS

Symptoms

In this condition, some of the tissue that normally lines the uterus (endometrium) "mislocates" and infiltrates other parts of the pelvic area—

on the ovaries, external surface of the uterus, ligaments or Fallopian tubes. Endometriosis can bring on severe pelvic pain around the time of menstruation and during ovulation and/or sexual activity; excessive or irregular menstrual flow, a higher-than-average rate of miscarriage; and infertility. Some women are completely unaware of the condition until they attempt to conceive and cannot. It is usually a painful condition caused by hormonal imbalance and is often aggravated by a stressful life. There may be painful intercourse, difficulties in bowel movements and urination.

Natural Remedies

While no single cause has been established, this disorder seems to be related to varying forms of tension. It is stress that can upset the body's delicate hormone balance. Normally, the progesterone produced at ovulation causes endometrial cells to die out. But women under stress do not ovulate at all; or do so sporadically, resulting in excess estrogen, providing a favorable environment for the growth of endometrial tissue.

Soothe that Stress! You need to control stress and unwind. Relaxation is helpful for pregnancy itself, often considered a cure for endometriosis in its mild form. Practice stress-management techniques. Switch jobs or relationships if they trigger chronic tension. Enjoy marital love for its own sake, not just to make babies. If you are trying too hard, you impose excessive pressure on yourself, which affects the sperm, too. In brief, focus on doing things that make you both emotionally and physically happy.

Vitamins May Ease Symptoms. Niels Lauersen, M.D., Professor of Obstetrics and Gynecology at Mt. Sinai Hospital, in New York City, feels nutrition should be considered as a remedy. "Endometriosis is such a terrible condition that every possible form of relief should be tried, while doctors make their determined efforts to eliminate the illness.

"We do know that certain vitamins may influence bodily functions. The B-complex vitamins, which affect neural transmissions that orchestrate menstrual flows, have been used to regulate periods. There have been cases of women who overcame endometriosis with high daily doses of vitamin B complex, vitamin E, and selenium.

"It is important for a woman to continue a health habit that works for her. Vitamins will not harm a woman with endometriosis, and although we do not have scientific proof that vitamins will cure the condition, maybe they will do some, as yet undocumented, good."[65]

Seafood May Ease Pain. Fish contains omega-3 fatty acids, which block production of pain-causing prostaglandins. You may want to prepare a chart. Note when your symptoms are worse as contrasted to when they are hardly noticeable. Then boost your intake of fish when you approach the painful time. Better yet, eat more fish throughout the month to regulate hormone balance to minimize discomfort all the time.

Warm Away the Pain. An old-time remedy for cramping and low back pain should help relieve pain of endometriosis. Apply a heating pad, moist heat to the cramping muscles of your abdomen. **TIP:** Increase intake of comfortably hot beverages for overall soothing comfort.

Can You Chill the Hurt? For some women, a cold pack is more beneficial than heat. Place an ice pack on your lower stomach area to numb the hurt.

Fitness Fades the Pain. Daily exercise helps reduce levels of estrogen, which slows the growth of endometriosis. Exercise boosts the manufacture of endorphins, those natural pain-blocking substances that make you feel glad all over. **CAREFUL:** Try gentle daily walking as an exercise; avoid too vigorous movements that can pull on scar tissue and adhesions.

Do-It-Yourself Acupressure. When you feel the onset of pain, you have two spots you can press gently—that's g–e–n–t–l–y—for soothing relief. (1) The inside of your leg, about two inches over your ankle bone. The right spot feels a bit sensitive. (2) The base where the bones of your thumb and index finger meet. *How to Do It*: Press either or both of these spots as hard as you comfortably can. Do **not** hurt yourself, since you want to ease the pain. This simple set of acupressure movements helps ease pain if repeated frequently. It works especially well if applied at the first start of pain.

EYES

Symptoms

Some physical changes occur during the normal aging process that can cause a gradual decline in vision. Older people generally need brighter light for such tasks as reading, cooking or driving a car. In addition, incandescent light bulbs (regular household bulbs) are better than fluorescent lights (tubular overhead lights) for older eyes. If you see halos around lights or flashes of light, if you have severe eye pain, if your vision is fading, if your eyes protrude or bulge, see your health practitioner without delay. With proper care, you can enjoy better vision no matter what your age.

Natural Remedies

For common and uncommon eye disorders, here is an assortment of helpful home remedies:

Black Eye. Symptom of tissue damage—typically from a blow to the eye area. Apply cold compresses to the injured eye to constrict blood vessels and then seek help from an ophthalmologist promptly since there may be internal bleeding.

Dark Circles. Delicate skin beneath your eyes may develop dark creases if you are overworked and abuse your sight with less sleep. These dark circles are small veins returning the blood to your heart. You may have an allergy that brings on the dark circles. Otherwise, be sure to get more rest. Sometimes, if you have lost weight too fast, the circles appear. Drink more liquids. Otherwise, you can hide them by wearing tinted glasses. The ladies have available special makeup to disguise the creases.

Dry Eyes. You feel burning, as if your eyeball is being swept by hot sand. Medically called *keratitis sicca,* dry eyes happens when there are changes in quality or quantity of tears produced by the tear glands. Without needed lubrication, the whites of your eyes become irritated, bloodshot and swollen. Check to see if you are allergic to something in the environment. Also, try specially formulated "artificial tears" in the form of a product. You apply some drops to help moisturize your scraping eyelids. **TIPS:** Use only white tissues if you must wipe your eyes. Try a humidifier at your work or living site. Wear sunglasses. Keep away from harsh chemicals with fumes that hurt your eyes. If you are taking medications, they could worsen the problem so discuss it with your doctor. In some situations, application of vitamin A directly to the eye stimulates the moisture-producing cells. This relieves symptoms and sensitivity. Your eyesight specialist can advise you on this method.

Eyelashes, Turning in. Called entropion, it occurs when the fibrous tissue on the lower lids becomes weak. There could also be a sagging lower lid (called ectropion), which is often irritating. To ease, attach one end of a piece of adhesive tape to the skin beneath your lower lashes. Tape the other end to your cheek. Let it remain for three days. Remove the tape to see if the condition has cleared up. Otherwise, see your eye doctor.

Eye Itching. Anxiety, allergy, eyestrain, neglected eye problem . . . any or all may cause itching. Apply warm or cold compresses to your closed eye to soothe the itch. Do **not** rub your eyes. Do **not** share tissues, handkerchief, or towels with anyone else, lest you spread an infection. **NEVER** patch the itching eye because the warm, enclosed eye could incubate bacteria!

Eye Puffiness. Fluid around and under the eyes collect to cause puffiness. During aging, the skin tends to lose its elasticity, and these surrounding tissues become more vulnerable to swelling or insistent gravity. Excessive drinking and tiredness worsens the disorder. **TIPS:** You want to distribute the blood, which you can do by remaining in an upright position, sitting, or standing. (If you scrub floors, do anything with your head held downward, such as sleeping, your blood is forced to move "uphill" to return to your heart, which increases the puffiness.) Keep your head held high! Wrap ice cubes in a cloth and apply to the region for quick relief. Sleep on your back instead of your stomach.

Floaters. Or "spots before the eyes" are tiny specks that float across your field of vision. You notice them in well-lighted rooms or outdoors on a bright day. Although normal and usually harmless, they may be a warning of certain eye problems, especially if associated with light flashes. **CAUTION:** if you notice a sudden change in the type or number of spots or flashes, see your doctor.

Eyestrain. Improve your focusing power with better illumination. Use a soft light that gives contrast, but not glare, when you read. Do not use any light that reflects directly back into your eyes as a mirror. Take a break from any close work (reading, sewing, computer operation, TV) every two hours . . . or more frequently. Do distant looking for a contrast. Of course, rest is an excellent way to ease eyestrain. Just close your eyes and relax! Massage your eyes—yes, you can do it by blinking your eyes 400 times a day. Each blink washes your eyes, refreshes them and actually massages them! Do this often!

Eyebright Tea. This herbal tea is said to help improve health of the eyes. You can also apply eyebright tea to your eyes. Soak a clean washcloth in freshly brewed eyebright tea. Lie down. Put the warm washcloth over your closed eyes and relax for 20 minutes. You will ease eyestrain. **CAREFUL:** Do not pour tea into your eyes; and the washcloth should be warm—never hot—when applied to your eyes!

Vitamins for Your Eyes. Suggestions are offered by Robert H. Garrison, Jr., Registered Pharmacist, and Elizabeth Somer, Registered Dietitian, from San Diego, California who tell us:

- *vitamin A*. Essential for normal development of eye tissue and vision. Retinol binds to a specialized eye protein to form rhodopsin, a molecule that helps you see in dim light. This vitamin is needed for development of epithelial tissues that line the eye.

- *vitamin B$_2$*. Needed to protect against vision loss, guard against burning and itching of the eyes. A deficiency of this vitamin is more prevalent in patients with cataracts than in healthy subjects.

- *vitamin B$_{12}$*. Increased intake will reverse poor vision if it results from inadequate dietary intake.

- *vitamin C*. Protects against cataracts. Galactose, a type of sugar, can produce cataracts in some people . . . and vitamin C helps build resistance to this disorder.

- *vitamin E*. An antioxidant that protects the polyunsaturated fats in epithelial cells lining the eye. Free radicals in air pollution, tobacco smoke and other environmental substances increase tissue damage if you have inadequate antioxidants. Vitamin E concentrations decrease in eye tissue during aging. This deficiency may bring on lipofuscin deposition in the pigmented epithelium of the retina and reduced visual acuity during aging.

- *Fish Oil*. Eicosapentaenoic acid (EPA) and other omega-3 fatty acids in fish oil enter the eye tissue and are believed to help protect against potentially permanent, partial loss of vision. Fish oils should be part of your natural remedy program for better sight.

- *Minerals*. Copper, chromium, zinc, magnesium are believed helpful in building resistance to cataracts.[66]

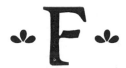

FEVER

Symptoms

A fever is your body's way of telling you that an infection is present. It is a defensive mechanism to combat this infection. A doctor should always be called if a fever suddenly changes from slight (99°F to 100°F) to high (104°F) and persists. Individual temperatures may vary throughout the day, running lower in the morning and higher in the evening. Slight changes in temperature (other than normal variation during the day) are usually not significant. A major increase in temperature (to approximately 104°F or over) may indicate a serious condition.

Natural Remedies

Fever is believed to be therapeutic and should be allowed to run its course. If it makes you miserable, try some of these helpful remedies:

Keep Yourself Liquefied. During a heated fever, your body perspires to cool you down. If you lose too much water, your body shuts off its sweat ducts to protect against more water loss. You may have difficulties because of this turn off process. All you need to do is drink lots of liquids . . . water is the mainstay. Sip liquids throughout the day.

Fruit and Vegetable Juices. They are rich in vitamins and minerals, which you lose during perspiration. Select a variety of such juices but avoid those that are high in sodium.

Cool Off with a Compress. Apply cool compresses to your forehead. When it becomes warm, remove the compress and apply a fresh one. Also apply to wrists and calves. (Keep the rest of your body covered.)

Soothing Sponge Bath. Evaporation cools your body and lowers the feverish temperature, but it also leaves wastes. Wring out a sponge, soak in cool tap water, wipe one section of your body at a time. Keep the rest of yourself covered. Pay special note to body regions which have the most heat: armpits and groin. No need to towel off because body heat will help moisture evaporate.

Alcohol Bath? Inadvisable. Alcohol evaporates more quickly than water and is not too soothing for a fever. There are the twin dangers of inhaling the vapors or absorbing them through pores.

Keep Yourself Comfortable. Feel overheated? Remove extra clothes so body heat can evaporate into the air. Feel chilly? Bundle up so you feel comfortable. A good household temperature is said to be about 65°F, not higher. Air should freely circulate. Keep out of drafts. Indirect lighting is soothing, which is relaxing.

Feed (or Starve) a Fever? Don't worry! Instead, drink more juices until the fever starts to reduce. Eat lightly as you recover. The choice is yours. If it helps you . . . do it! More important, you have an increased demand for liquids.

A set of home remedies is offered by Dr. Varro E. Tyler, a pharmacognosist with Purdue University:

- To reduce a fever, drink tea made from the feverfew herb.
- Drink hot ginger tea to break a high fever.
- An excellent fever drink is made from the juice of one lemon, one teaspoonful of cream of tartar, and one pint of water, sweetened to taste. Drink freely when thirsty.
- Drink spicebush tea to cool a fever.

These herbs are available at most health food stores and herbal pharmacies.[67]

Quick-Acting Fever Remedies. Folk healers include:

- Take hot lemon and honey as often as desired because lemon has antibacterial benefits.
- Take frequent drinks of elderflower, peppermint, or yarrow tea to promote perspiration and reduce temperature.
- Elderflower is also useful for reducing any nasal inflammation. If this is accompanied by a penetrating chill, add grated ginger root or cayenne.
- Black pepper sprinkled over food also has a restorative effect, or you could take an infusion of mustard seed, ¼ teaspoon powder infused for five minutes in one cup of boiling water. Repeat three times a day.

FIBROSITIS

Symptoms

Inflammation of the fibrous connective tissue, especially an acute inflammation of back muscles and their sheaths, causing pain and stiffness. This is a common condition that may not be a specific disease. Tests may reveal no signs of damage to the structures. Some doctors do not use the term "fibrositis" for such symptoms but call it and similar conditions: muscular rheumatism, musculoskeletal pain syndrome, nonarticular rheumatism, or fibromyalgia. The muscles become tight and tense; you may feel emotionally and physically drained. You may have very tender "trigger points" over your shoulders, back, hips, and in certain other body areas. *Note:* Fibrositis is a condition in which deep sleep is unattainable. It afflicts tense, perfectionist-type people. For them, the norm is shallow sleep that gives rise to muscle spasms and pain in various body parts called "tender body spots."

Natural Remedies

Your first step is to "give it a rest." You will help cool off the inflammation and stiffness with less pressure. You will also find relief by taking a whirlpool bath. Or else, a soak in warm water helps speed up blood flow.

Stretching gently is a soothing way to limber up gnarled muscles. Do this easily so that you do not hurt your overworked muscles.

Put The Pain on Ice. Wrap ice cubes in a clean cloth and apply to the hurt area for 15 minutes. Repeat as often as desired. Or else, wrap a small can of frozen food in the cloth and let its coolness take the heat off your pain.

Change Your Position. If you keep joints or muscles in the same position for a long time, you increase painful stiffness. For example, writing a long letter keeps your hand in the same position for as long as it takes to finish the letter. TIP: Relax and stretch your hand and arm every five minutes or so.

Use Stronger Joints and Muscles. Whenever possible, follow these pressure-easing guidelines:

• Carry a purse over your shoulder on a strap, rather than holding it in your hand. It has less pressure!

- Push open a heavy door with the side of your arm, not with your hand and outstretched arm.
- When lifting something that is low or on the ground, bend your knees and lift with your back straight.
- Spread the weight of an object over many joints to reduce stress placed on one joint.
- Using a firm mattress or a board between your mattress and box spring will help you keep correct posture while you sleep or rest in bed. Changes in sitting posture are especially important if you sit at work or home for long periods. Make sure you do not slump.
- Footwear is important for posture. High heels put more stress on lower backs than low or flat heels do. Your shoes should be strong enough to provide support for your feet and prevent your legs from tiring.

Ease that Stress. Fibrositis flares up when you are subjected to stress. Following relaxation exercises helps your back muscles relax so that pain can be reduced. Pace yourself during the day and also from day to day. Allow yourself plenty of time to finish the things you start so you won't feel rushed. Balance rest with activity!

Laugh It Off. Laughter may fight pain and inflammatory conditions because it stimulates your brain to produce catecholamines, also known as the "alertness hormones." These hormones trigger the release of the brain's natural pain killers, endorphins. So . . . enjoy a healthy dose of laughter.

CASE HISTORY—*Sends Near-Crippling Fibrositis into Remission . . . Naturally*

Years of wear and tear on his shoulder and middle-back muscles gave George Q. a painful case of fibrositis. As a warehouse supervisor, he needed to keep physically active . . . and soon found the shooting muscle spasms doubled him over with agonizing pain. He could scarcely move a small wagon or carton of merchandise. George Q. tried medications which dulled the pain . . . and when the drugs wore off, the pain returned with an angry vengeance! He faced being crippled, until a physiatrist (specialist in rehabilitation treatment) put him on an exercise program, told him how to lift properly, how to ease stress and join humor groups and laugh more. In six weeks, George Q. was able to send the near-crippling fibrositis into remission . . . naturally!

FINGERNAILS

Symptoms

Like hair, your nails are composed of a tough protein called keratin that is formed by the nail matrix, a specialized group of cells beneath the base of the nail. Part of the matrix is usually visible as the lunula, or half-moon, at the base of the thumb nail.

The matrix and nail bed are living tissues located beneath the nail plate, as the nail itself is called. A normal nail bed appears pink through the nail plate, a reflection of a healthy underlying blood supply. By looking at nails, doctors can detect signs of malnutrition, carpal tunnel syndrome, stress injury, and various other illnesses. Typical symptoms and possible disorders seen by looking at nails include:

Red Streaks. High blood pressure, ulcers.

Pitting. Eczema, psoriasis, among other problems.

Yellow Nails. Diseases of the thyroid and lymph system cause nails to become thick, rough and yellow; chronic respiratory disease, long-term use of tetracycline.

Blue Color. If the nail bed or lunula appears blue, there may be circulatory disorders caused by heart trouble, diabetes or Raynaud's disease (spasms of arteries in the fingers because of cold).

Spoon Nails. Are your nail plates spoonlike or depressed? Symptomatic of anemia or thyroid disease.

Horizontal Furrows. Also known as Beau's lines across the nail plate. May result from serious illness, carpal tunnel syndrome, or malnutrition.

Clubbing. An upwardly raised curve and the curling of the nails around the fingertips may indicate disorders of the heart, colon, liver, lungs.

White Streaks. Also known as Mee's lines, if they go down the length of the nail, there could be heart trouble, kidney failure, Hodgkin's disease, or reactions to treatment with cancer drugs.

Splinter Hemorrhages. Red streaks going down the length of the nail bed might suggest hypertension, rheumatoid arthritis, ulcers, endocarditis, psoriasis.

Onycholysis. Separation of the nail plate from the nail bed. May be caused by psoriasis, fungal infection, or systemic disorders, such as hyperthyroidism. Trauma on the nail plate and reactions to certain drugs, such as formalin (commercial nail hardener), could cause separation.

Brittle Nails. Fraying or peeling of the ends of the nails. Often the result of household damage from the use of detergents and alkalis; Cold weather or lack of moisture causes the horny layer to become dry and brittle. Excessive manicuring, a reaction to a solvent used in nail polish and lacquer may be a reason for brittleness.

Natural Remedies

For strong fingernails, take better care of your overall health and try these remedies:

- To counteract brittleness, soak your nails in warm olive oil for 10 to 15 minutes each day.
- For fragile nails that break and split (when not caused by disease), protect them with several coats of nail polish. **CAREFUL:** Clipping or extreme filing, especially when the nails are filed to a point or a triangular shape, may weaken the nail corners or make the edges fragile.
- Wear gloves whenever possible during activities that might injure your nails or fingertips or overexpose them to the elements.
- After your hands have been in water, apply a moisturizing lotion (one that contains a minimum of 10 percent urea), and rub the lotion on the nail plate, as well as into the surrounding soft tissue.
- Nail polish offers temporary strength to weak nails, but it will dry them, and excessive use of nail polish remover will cause splitting. Instead, avoid removing polish more than once every two weeks. Touch up chips, instead.
- Instead of polish, buff your nails so they become shiny-smooth. Avoid overusing buffing compounds which may thin your nails.

- Manicure fingernails with a flexible emery board; leave a small amount of white nail visible at the corners. If a cuticle tears, trim it promptly with a sharp cuticle scissors; be careful not to pull away parts that are firmly attached. **TIP:** Cuticles protect your nail matrix from attack by infectious organisms or damaging chemicals, so let them remain attached to the nail plate.

- Stay away from polishes that contain formaldehyde. So-called oily polish remover could be hurtful. To restore moisture to your nails and surrounding skin, soak them in warm water a few minutes, pat them dry, then rub in olive oil, petroleum jelly, emollient cream or moisturizer with a lanolin base.

- Artificial nails are dangerous! They are made of highly allergenic plastics and applied with similarly allergenic adhesives. If a reaction occurs in the nail bed, the whole nail may fall out!

- Nail hardeners and fortifiers are temporary. Hardeners actually dehydrate your nails and provide no more extra strength than is available from one coat of polish.

- Cuticle removers have their risks. They expose your nails to possible infection. Do **NOT** push cuticles back to the bottom of the nail because this will break the protective seal between skin and nail. **TIP:** If you have a hangnail, cut if off with a sharp scissors, but be careful not to dig into and injure the live tissue to which it is attached.

- Since nails are most brittle when dry, cut them when wet to eliminate breakage.

- Use an emery board to smooth and sand the surface of nails, especially near the edges. This eliminates defects that allow breaks and splits.

- Weak and brittle nails can sometimes be helped by painting transparent or "white" iodine under them and also around the cuticles.

- Avoid putting your hands into very hot water and/or detergents if at all possible because they dry your nails. **TIP:** If your hands are immersed in water a great deal, apply some anti-wet barrier cream into all the crevices around the nails for protection.

- Lemon juice is a useful nail cleanser; it is a good idea to keep a slice of lemon near your kitchen sink for this purpose after household chores. And . . . while your brittle nails are improving, wear a pair of rubber gloves temporarily to speed the healing process.

- Run your fingernails along your palm when washing your hands to force the soapy lather under your nails. This cleans away germ-breeding dirt.

- Fungus infections around the nails are most distressing. Oral antibiotics destroy valuable intestinal bacteria and can cause such infections to develop not only internally but also in the fingers and under the nails. **TIP:** Daily intake of yogurt or acidophilus milk helps restore intestinal flora. Vitamin B complex is also helpful.

Good basic care of your fingers (and hands) includes protection against irritants and overdrying. Wear rubber gloves with cotton liners while doing wet work. Protect your hands with gloves or mittens during cold weather. Lubricate your hands, especially the cuticles, with an emollient cream daily, or several times a day if necessary. Do not bite, chew, clip, or push the cuticles or surrounding tissue. If you must clip cuticles, clip more often, a little at a time, instead of cutting too much in one session. Always use clean instruments for cuticle and nail care.

FLU

Symptoms

Also known as influenza, flu is a viral infection that is quite common during the winter season. The most common symptoms include a feeling of being utterly miserable; there is fever (sometimes with chills), cough, muscle aches, fatigue, and a general feeling of illness. There may also be a sore throat, nasal discharge, headaches, and loss of appetite. The worst symptoms usually subside after a few days, but there is a lingering feeling of tiredness for a week or so. **CAUTION:** Flu is contagious. The infection is transmitted by respiratory secretions that become airborne during coughing and sneezing. Thus, close contact with a person with influenza who is coughing or sneezing is likely to result in infection. **DANGER:** If one person in a household has flu, the rest of the family may contract the condition—and it spreads rapidly through offices, classrooms, work sites. Symptoms usually develop 24 to 48 hours after exposure to the virus and the patient is contagious for three to four days after the onset of symptoms.

Natural Remedies

Basic treatment calls for these basics: Maintain a well-balanced diet with plenty of fluids. Be sure to get lots of bed rest and avoid cigarette smoking. Extra fluids call for at least one full glass every hour.

Avoid crowds. Since the virus spreads speedily, keep away from crowded areas (shopping centers, theatres, malls, etc.). And keep your distance from those you see sneezing or coughing . . . even if it means changing your seat on the commuter bus or train or getting off the elevator on the wrong floor.

Boost immunity by avoiding exposure to wet and/or cold weather. Dress warmly if you must face these elements.

Salt Water Gargle. You need relief and also want to wash out the wastes that are gathering in your throat. Properly mixed salt water is soothing. Gargle with a half teaspoon of salt mixed in a quart of lukewarm water. It bathes your mouth, helps wash away some bacteria, infected material and pus, which causes discomfort. **TIP:** Add a bit of baking soda to the solution to help break up thick mucus, to oxygenate your mouth and make it less friendly to bacteria.

Humidify Your Room. You'll ease discomfort of a cough, sore throat, or dry nasal passages. Ease chest congestion with a humidifier or vaporizer in your room.

Try a Hot Soak. Not your entire body—but you will ease headache and nasal congestion by soaking your feet in *comfortably* hot water. Add fragrant herbs to give you a nice feeling.

Ventilation Is Important. Your sickroom or living/working space should have a good supply of fresh air at all times. Keep out of drafts and chills, though. Protect yourself with warm, close-fitting garments.

Nutritional Flu-Busters. You need lots of liquids to overcome the dehydration caused by a fever. Can't eat? No appetite? Try thin soups, fruit and vegetable juices (rich in nutrients you lose during the illness). **TIP:** Dilute fruit juice equally with water, to provide a small amount of glucose, needed to give you energy; careful, too much sugar can cause diarrhea during the illness! Try any sugar-free soft drinks (avoid those with chemical sweeteners). Allow them to go flat before drinking, because their bubbles can create stomach gas and more nausea. When your appetite returns, try dry toast, bananas, boiled brown rice, cooked whole grain cereal, baked potatoes, applesauce, non-fat plain yogurt to which you may add pureed fruit.

FOOD POISONING OR SALMONELLA

Symptoms

So you have an "upset stomach." Or abdominal cramps. Or diarrhea. Or all three. Do you accept it as "one of those bugs going around?" In a way, you're right. These symptoms can be caused by any number of "bugs" or bacteria. So can many other symptoms. What you need to know is that many illnesses are caused by harmful bacteria in foods—and you may have a case of salmonella or botulism—or food poisoning! The bacteria that commonly cause poisoning—with mild-to-severe intestinal flu-like symptoms—are not obvious. Most cannot be seen, smelled, or tasted. To protect against such disorders, you need to play it safe in buying, handling, and cooking food. Beginning right away, make it a habit to follow a set of safety rules.

Natural Remedies

Prevent food contamination with these guidelines:

1. Clean your hands before and after handling raw foods. Wash thoroughly all cutting surfaces and utensils after each use.

2. Put perishable and frozen foods in your refrigerator as soon as you get home after shopping.

3. If you prepare foods ahead of time, put them in your refrigerator until you are ready to serve them.

4. Don't leave leftover foods on the table; store them in your refrigerator promptly.

5. Don't let frozen foods thaw at room temperature. Defrost them in your refrigerator.

6. Cool foods promptly in small quantities and in shallow layers, so that the temperature of the food is brought down to refrigerator temperature (40°F) in two to three hours.

7. When cooking meats, use a meat thermometer to make sure the interior part of the meat is cooked thoroughly (for example, at least 175°F to 185°F for poultry, 170°F for fresh meat).

8. If you do home canning, use the "cold pack" method for acid foods only. **TIP:** When canning non-acid foods, such as meats or vegetables, you cannot be sure that temperatures used in the "cold pack" method are high enough to kill the bacteria

that may cause botulism. **CAREFUL:** If you find a jar or can in which the food does not appear or smell right, destroy the entire lot. Do **not** taste the food. It could be fatal.

9. Be careful in the handling of pets in your home. Pet feeding dishes, toys or bedding should not be allowed in your kitchen or near any items that come in contact with the family's food, or with utensils or working surfaces used in the preparation of food.

10. One of the best ways to control bacterial contamination in food is by cooking at high temperatures. Extreme heat kills bacteria that might cause poisoning. High heat is especially necessary when preparing such foods as milk, milk products, eggs, **meat,** poultry, fish, and shellfish.

WARNING: Never store food in plastic bread bags! Do not recycle bread's plastic packaging to wrap sandwiches—small amounts of dangerous lead from the paint on the wrapper can get into the food. You may be tempted to turn the bags inside out and reuse them to store food. **DON'T DO IT!** This is a hazard—it allows paint to come into direct contact with food.

Beware: External printing contains some toxic lead, but it does not leak through the plastic and is allowed to be used. But . . . if you turn the bag inside out to remove crumbs or dry out the bag, the paint can come off and get into the food. Avoid this threat of lead exposure. Discard bread bags. Lead is especially dangerous for youngsters because it **inter**feres with the development of the nervous system.

Basic Remedies for Food Illness. For mild illness, treat symptoms much like "flu." Keep up your liquid intake with water, tea, apple juice, bouillon, and club soda to replace fluids lost through diarrhea or vomiting. For severe symptoms, or if the victim is very young, elderly or has **a** chronic illness, seek medical care promptly.

Don't Interfere with Nature. Your body wants to wash out infectious organisms, so don't interfere with this cleansing. If you take antidiarrheal products, you could block your body's ability to fight the infection. If you insist on a medication, consult your health practitioner.

De-Fizz Soft Drinks. Flat soft drinks are soothing to your intestinal tract and replace lost fluid. Best to avoid regular soft drinks because the carbonation can cause further irritation. De-fizzed soft drinks help settle your stomach. Refreshing, too!

FUNGAL INFECTION

Symptoms

Fungal infections include candidiasis, urinary tract infection, more familiar athlete's foot, pneumonia, "jock itch," to name a few. Although harmless for most of the population, fungal infections can be fatal in those with impaired immune defense mechanisms, particularly cancer patients, burn victims, transplant recipients, diabetics, patients on long-term antibiotic therapy and people with AIDS. Fungi may enter the body and depress the immune system by way of inhalation and breaks in the skin. The familiar "itch" whether on the feet or groin, or elsewhere, is a typical symptom. Once in the body, the fungi organisms may migrate to any part of the body, overpower lymphocytes and pass through tissue into the bloodstream, making any organ vulnerable to attack.

Natural Remedies

Fungal infections of the skin, hair and nails are among the most frequently occurring skin diseases. "The majority of fungal infections treated by dermatologists are not life-threatening," says Jack L. Lesher, Jr., M.D., associate Professor of Dermatology at the Medical College of Georgia in Atlanta. "But the quality of life can be significantly diminished."

Sneaker Foot. "This can initially appear as redness and scaling of the feet which later develop into blistering, crusting and oozing," explains Dr. Lesher. "The combination of sneakers, feet in confinement and perspiration creates the right environment for this condition." *Remedy*: "Wear white cotton socks and change them frequently. Use a moisturizing lotion on any dry skin. Avoid sneakers for a period of time."

Ringworm of the Scalp. Also known as *tinea capitis,* "it has nothing to do with worms. In more severe cases, there can be thickened scaling and even hair loss. Combs, brushes and hats should never be shared. It's a good idea to check the family pet who can either be a carrier or infected with the fungus." *Remedy*: "It does not respond to topical creams or shampoos, but a medicated shampoo can cut down on the infectious scale. Any infected children should be kept out of school while treatment is started since ringworm is contagious," advises Dr. Lesher.[68]

Keep Feet Warm and Dry. Feet damp and chilled after being outdoors? Indoors, get out of those shoes and socks. Dry feet thoroughly (especially between toes and nails) to prevent any foot fungus from taking hold. Moisture on the feet causes the same effect as sprinklers on on the lawn. Something will grow—but is it something you want?

Jock Itch. Remedies are offered by Donald M. Vickery, M.D., and James F. Fries, M.D., authors of *Take Care Of Yourself.* "Jock itch or *tinea cruris* is a fungal infection of the pubic region. It is aggravated by friction and moisture. It usually does not involve the scrotum or penis, nor does it spread beyond the groin area. For the most part, this is a male disease. Frequently, the fungus grows in an athletic supporter turned old and moldy in a locker room far from a washing machine. The preventive measure for such a problem is obvious."

Home Treatment. Drs. Vickery and Fries suggest, "The problem should be treated by removing the contributing factors—friction and moisture. This is done by wearing boxer-type shorts rather than closer-fitting shorts, by applying a powder to dry the area after bathing. Make frequent changes of soiled or sweaty underclothes. It may take up to two weeks to completely clear the problem, and it may recur. The 'powder-and-clean-shorts' treatment will usually be successful without any medication."[69]

Heal Your Chapped Hands. Splits and cracks on your hands may look chapped . . . but if they do not heal up within two weeks, you may have a fungal infection. Anyone (medical people, kitchen workers, housewives) who constantly immerse hands in water can easily contract *monilial paronychia,* an annoying fungal infection involving skin around the cuticle. When the infection strikes the finger's protective nail fold, it becomes swollen, red, painful. The danger is that the fungal infection may spread to other body parts that come in contact with your hands . . . and it is prudent to try speedy remedies very quickly.

Vegetable Shortening Is Soothing. Ordinary vegetable shortening helps heal chapped skin. It's a wonderful moisturizer that covers the skin and locks in water. Use *very little* and rub it thoroughly so your hands do not feel greasy. You may also use cocoa butter, lanolin, light mineral oil, petroleum oil.

Citrus Oil Rub. Mix a few drops of glycerin (from any pharmacy) with a few drops of lemon oil (from any pharmacy) and rub into your chapped skin at bedtime. This citrus oil rub will moisturize and heal your chapped skin . . . while you sleep.

Take a Salt Soak. To nip a fungal infection in the bud anywhere on your body, take a salt bath. Add one cup of ordinary salt to an average tub of warm water. Soak in this salt bath for about 15 minutes. Do this twice a day. The saline solution discourages the fungus, controls perspiration, soothes the affected skin.

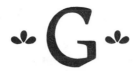

GALLBLADDER

Symptoms

The gallbladder is a small pear-shaped organ tucked under the liver, where it serves as a storage site for bile, a fluid essential to the digestion of fatty foods. Trouble hits in the form of gallstones, which are clumps of solid material usually made of either cholesterol or bile. Gallstones can be as small as a grain of sand or as big as an egg. The gallbladder may develop into a single, often large, stone or many smaller ones, even several thousand. **DANGER:** Small stones can move into the bile ducts and become lodged there, blocking the flow of bile and causing pain and jaundice. Larger stones can block the outlet from the gallbladder and cause steady, sharp pain when the gallbladder tries to empty. The people most likely to develop gallstones are women who have been pregnant; overweight people who eat a lot of dairy products and animal fats; and people over 60. Look for these warning signs:

- severe and steady pain in the upper abdomen, which can spread to the chest, shoulders or back, and is sometimes mistaken for the symptoms of a heart attack.
- indigestion, nausea or vomiting.
- severe abdominal pain and tenderness in the right side of the abdomen when the gallbladder is inflamed.
- jaundice, chills, and fever when gallstones block the passage of bile. (Jaundice is a yellow discoloration of the skin and eyes.)

Natural Remedies

Surgery is a common method for treating gallstones by removing the gallbladder. But not all people are good candidates for surgery, either because they may be too weak or they have another medical condition that greatly increases the risks involved. Consider alternatives to surgery.

Keep Fat Intake to a Minimum. In some studies, vegetarian women—who eat less saturated fat and no meat but have a high fiber intake—had one-half the incidence of gallstones. Fat reduction in the diet may help build resistance to gallstone formation.

Lecithin: The Food that Protects Against Gallstones. Lecithin is a food derived from soybeans or the sunflower plant. It is a phospholipid (fat-dissolving) food that increases elimination of fatty compounds from the body. Lecithin contains phosphatidylcholine which emulsifies cholesterol, makes fat more soluble and less likely to form into gallstones. Lecithin granules are available at most health stores. Easy to use in your morning cereal for added fiber to keep your gallbladder clean and free of fat.

Lose Dangerous Overweight. Limit your intake of fatty foods and lose that overweight. The reason is that fats need bile in order to be absorbed. The gallbladder must contract to push the bile into the intestine, whereupon pain is caused by the blocked outlet. With less fat and obesity, there is less vulnerability to attack.

CASE HISTORY—*Loses Fatty Weight and "Loses" Gallstones*

Joan H. complained of abdominal pain and bouts of nausea. Her internist diagnosed jaundice as a symptom of gallbladder trouble and the potential for gallstones. She was not a candidate for surgery which she wanted to avoid because of certain risks involved concerning another condition. Her internist chose an alternative route. Joan H. was put on a fat-lowering program that helped melt away excess weight. Her cholesterol-triglyceride levels also dropped to a more healthful level. She was told to eat at least six to eight tablespoons of lecithin daily in her high-fiber cereal, with non-fat milk or natural fruit juice. *Benefit*: lecithin functioned as a "detergent" by dissolving fats and water-soluble wastes at the same time. She was told to boost intake of fresh fruit juices because the vitamin C would work with lecithin to process cholesterol so it could be washed out via the bile salts. *Results*: Joan H. was saved from surgery when the fat-reduction, lecithin-washing, vitamin C-cleansing program helped her "lose" the gallstones. Gone was the pain, too! She calls lecithin and vitamin C her "gallbladder cleansers!"

GASTRITIS

Symptoms

A common stomach disorder, it has two levels.

1. Acute gastritis is an inflammation of the lining of the stomach. It may be caused by excessive alcohol, food poisoning, or a bacterial infection. An attack may be triggered by drugs, such as aspirin or anti-arthritic medications. Symptoms include abdominal pain and tenderness, loss of appetite, nausea and vomiting.

2. Chronic gastritis occurs when the symptoms persist for a long period of time. There may be an invasion of bacteria that has infected the stomach lining. This occurs frequently with aging, but may be associated with other disorders, such as chronic stomach ulcers or a vitamin B_{12} deficiency.

Natural Remedies

Remake your digestive system with a rejuvenating program that calls for these methods:

- Easy does it with alcohol. If possible, eliminate entirely for the sake of a healthier digestive system.
- Cool off the inflammation by controlling heated stress—it can set off a chain reaction to upset your stomach lining.
- Do not eat too much . . . and do **not** eat too quickly!
- Avoid foods and beverages containing caffeine, which may lead to inflammation of the stomach lining.
- If you have an acute attack, go on an immediate fast for at least one day to give your stomach a chance to cool off. Stick to room-temperature water. After this one day fast, gradually introduce bland foods to coax your digestive system into contented healing.
- Keep away from irritants: salt, pepper, strong spices, highly acidic foods.
- Avoid high-fat foods because they slow the rate at which food moves through your digestive system and cause distress.
- Avoid smoking . . . and people who smoke because the sidestream can be as hurtful as if you smoked a cigarette yourself!
- If the gastritis can be linked to a particular offending food, then merely eliminate that source.

Vitamin B_{12} Is Healing to Stomach Lining. In chronic gastritis, there is cellular destruction in the stomach lining, with poor absorption of vitamin B_{12}. A deficiency will worsen the condition. To protect against such problems, be sure to boost intake of foods containing this vitamin:

cooked lean beef, chicken, fish, liver (careful, high in cholesterol), and cooked whitefish. The only plant able to synthesize vitamin B_{12} is the leafy green vegetable, comfrey. Small amounts of these foods will help restore the health of your stomach lining and ease chronic gastritis.

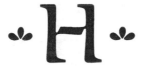

HAIR AND SCALP

Symptoms

Most scalp hair loss is normal. Adults have approximately 100,000 hairs on their heads. These hairs follow a very predictable pattern of active growing (about 90 percent of hair at any one time), followed by a resting and shedding period (about 10 percent of hair). The growth period may last as long as two to ten years, whereas the resting/shedding stage may take only a few months. On average, you lose and replace about 50 to 150 hairs per day. Hair grows slightly faster in women than men. Visible hair loss occurs when the number of hairs in the growth phase no longer keeps pace with the number of hairs in the shedding stage. Men tend to lose hair around the front of the face and the crown (or "vertex") of the scalp. Hair loss in women tends to appear as overall thinning.

Hormones are thought to play a key role in scalp hair growth and loss. It's known, for example, that while testosterone and other androgens are largely responsible for the growth of body hair at puberty, these same androgens are key to hair loss in adults. Many birth control pills are androgen dominant and can spur hair loss. It is believed that estrogen helps to curb scalp hair loss and encourage healthy scalp hair growth. The process is not only hormonal, but may also be related to other substances in the blood that go to hair follicles. In some people, various minerals may be involved because minerals are part of the enzymatic system that affects hair growth, health, and loss.

Natural Remedies

If you treat it kindly, your hair can surely become your crowning glory. Current practices of bleaching, rolling, and dyeing tend to torture your hair and scalp, causing deleterious reactions. Put health back into your hair with a program of natural care and helpful remedies.

Dandruff. The "snow on your shoulders" is a normal process of shedding dead cells to make way for new ones. Flakes of old cells become trapped in your hair shafts and are visible as small white scales. **CAREFUL:** Dandruff may be triggered by stress, hormonal changes, and poor diet that has devitalized foods and refined sugars and starches. If you're itching to get to the root of this head-scratching problem, try natural remedies.

Shampoo Regularly. It becomes easier to control dandruff with frequent shampoos. Try a product that contains selenium sulfide or zinc pyrithione because these ingredients control the rate at which scalp cells multiply. *Old-fashioned tar shampoo.* It works! Lather with tar shampoo and let it remain on scalp for 10 minutes. The tar will help penetrate your shaft and cleanse the follicle so you will be able to wash out your pesky dandruff. If a tar shampoo is a bit too harsh at the start, alternate with your regular shampoo. **TIP:** Be sure to lather twice . . . and then rinse very thoroughly under a tepid shower.

Herbal Shampoo. Boil four heaping tablespoons of dried thyme in two glasses of water for 10 minutes. Strain. Let it cool. Pour the mixture over clean damp hair. Massage your scalp with your fingertips to loosen scales and flakes. Do **NOT** scratch your scalp or you will create sores that are more distressing than the dandruff. Then let it remain for 60 minutes. Wash off beneath free flowing tepid water. You'll have a dandruff-clear scalp and better color, too, because of the thyme.

Oil Improves Scalp Health. An occasional warm-oil home remedy helps soften and loosen clinging dandruff scales. Heat two tablespoons of olive oil on the stove until just warm. (Takes only a minute or two.) Pre-wet your hair (or else the oil will be soaked into your hair instead of getting to your scalp). Dip a soft brush or cotton ball into the oil and apply directly to your scalp. Section your hair to reach your scalp. Put on a shower cap and let the oil remain for 30 minutes. Then wash out the oil with a dandruff shampoo. Do this once a week and you'll improve your dandruff-infested scalp!

Home Made Dandruff Cleaning Shampoo. Beat the yolks of two eggs in a half cup of warm water. Massage gently into your hair and scalp for five to ten minutes. Rinse carefully. Finish with a rinse of two teaspoons of apple cider vinegar mixed in water. Towel-dry your hair.

Dry Hair. Excessive shampooing and swimming will lead to dry hair, along with chemical colorants, electric curlers, excessive blow-drying, harsh exposure to sun and wind, salty, chlorinated or sudsy water may also be to blame. How to save your dried-out tresses that are limp and unmanageable? Try these remedies.

Give Your Hair a Shampoo Break. Wash hair less often; select a mild shampoo or one made specifically "for dry or damaged hair."

Mayonnaise Conditioner. In dry hair, the cuticles (outer layers) separate from the main shaft. Conditioners fasten the cuticles back to the shaft, lubricate your tresses, protect against the frizzies (static electricity.) All you need do is apply ordinary mayonnaise to your hair and let it remain from 30 to 60 minutes so the ingredients nourish your scalp and help "glue" the cuticles back to the shaft. Wash off thoroughly.

Avoid Soap on Your Hair. Typical soap leaves an insoluble alkaline film on your scalp to clog your hair and oil openings and bring on drying and dandruff. Soap has an alkaline quality that removes the natural acid mantle of a healthy scalp and opens the way to bacterial invasion. **TIP:** Choose an egg or herbal shampoo for healthier crowning tresses.

Avocado Conditioner. This fruit is rich in many vitamins, minerals, and essential fatty acids that nourish your scalp. Massage a finely mashed avocado pulp into your hair and scalp for five minutes. Cover with a plastic bag; tuck in ends so you have scalp warmth. Let it remain for 60 minutes to penetrate your follicles. Then shampoo out with a non-alkaline product. **TIP:** Finish with a rinse of two teaspoons of lemon juice (for light-haired people) or two teaspoons of apple cider vinegar (for dark-haired people) to one quart of water.

Oily Hair. Each hair strand has its base firmly encased within the follicle or scalp opening, which also contains an opening from the sebaceous gland. This oil gland provides lubrication for your hair shaft and skin. But sometimes this "oil factory" does not know when to stop and the sebaceous gland becomes overly productive. You have oily hair! To control this outpouring, try some remedies.

Shampoo Is Needed. Summer heat and humidity stimulate your oil glands so shampoo more often. While you shampoo, massage your scalp to squeeze out some more oil. You may want to leave the shampoo on your oily hair for five minutes so the ingredients can penetrate and get the oil out. Do this twice during a single shampoo.

Lemon Rinse. Squeeze the juice of two lemons into one quart of distilled water (preferable because it works best). Use some as a rinse to help cut the oiliness.

Vinegar Rinse. One tablespoon of apple cider vinegar in one pint of water makes a great finishing rinse. Helps nourish your scalp and also removes soap goo that otherwise weighs down oily hair.

Which Shampoo? A natural shampoo is best . . . but it should be clear. If you can see through the shampoo, it will clean away the oil much better, and will not leave any residue behind.

Quick Herbal Shampoo. Pour one application of a mild baby shampoo into a cup and add two tablespoons of a herb (parsley, mint, rosemary, thyme, chamomile, comfrey, sage). Mix together and use in your typical manner.

HAY FEVER

Symptoms

Seasonal allergic rhinitis (more commonly known as hay fever) is an allergic response to pollen generated by trees, grasses or weeds. It is characterized by an itchy, runny, sneezy or stuffy nose; you may also have itchy, scratchy eyes. Ragweed pollen is the major culprit in most situations. It is windborne and finds you in almost any region. There are many other weeds that can cause pollen allergy, depending upon your region of the country and the particular season as you can see from the following chart.

Seasons	East and Midwest	South and South Central	West
SPRING	Tree pollen: oak, sycamore, birch	Tree pollen	Tree pollen
SUMMER	Grass pollen: blue-grass, redtop	Grass pollen	Grass pollen
FALL	Ragweed pollen In August and Sept. a quarter of a million tons of pollen blow through the Midwest.	Grass pollen Ragweed pollen	Tumbleweed and sage pollen
WINTER		Tree pollen Grass pollen	Tumbleweed and sage pollen

Seasons	East and Midwest	South and South Central	West
YEAR-ROUND	Mold spores on soil and vegetation are spread from April through November and trigger severe allergic reactions. Frost does not kill them.	In central Florida the ragweed season runs from June to November.	Because of lower ragweed pollen levels and higher elevations, the area in general offers sufferers a respite from seasonal allergies. Mold spores decrease at high altitudes and in dry areas.

Source: The American Academy of Allergy and Immunology

The weather does have some influence on hay fever symptoms. Days that are rainy, cloudy or windless serve to alleviate the condition because pollen is not disseminated as readily during these times. The return of hot, dry and windy weather will signal a return of pollen and mold distribution and discomfort.

Natural Remedies

Arthur M. Lubitz, M.D., Clinical Instructor on allergies and pulmonary specialist, with New York Medical College in New York City, has these suggestions:

1. Become a pollen expert. Learn when and where pollens are most prevalent. The chart is helpful but it does not replace a visit to a qualified allergist. Don't guess about the source of your symptoms.

2. Chill your allergies. Air-conditioning is one of the best ways to lessen allergen exposure. Central systems work best. Keep air-conditioning set at the highest comfortable setting—not lower than 70°F. TIP: If you're not at home, do not leave your air conditioner on, since it tends to pull in daytime pollen. Be sure to clean your air filter or wash it at least once a month.

3. Catch a sea breeze. Wind blowing in from the ocean is refreshing as long as it does not pass over a land mass before reaching you. CAREFUL: Air blowing out to sea is some of the most allergen-laden. DANGER: Beach weather—a hot sun and a strong breeze will give you a schnozola full of allergens.

4. Take advantage of summer showers since they wash pollen out of the air. TIP: If you're mold-allergic, your symptoms may be

worse right after several days of showers, since humidity promotes mold growth.

5. Keep away from liquor. Alcoholic beverages increase the severity of allergic reactions in some people, especially when the air is thick with allergens. Wine and beer are the worst offenders.

6. You may have an allergy to some foods. If you are allergic to ragweed you may have a cross-reaction with a variety of botanically similar species. These include watermelon and mangoes. If you have a reaction after eating any such fruits . . . avoid them during the season.

7. Don't dive or swim underwater. Swelling inside the ears is a common allergic symptom. The stress and pressure changes that accompany diving into the water can greatly aggravate ears, which pop or feel plugged because of allergen exposure.

8. Whether or not you're lactose intolerant, i.e., allergic to dairy products, if you're allergy-prone, cut down on dairy foods.[70]

Hints, Tips, Suggestions. Ease distress with these remedies:
—Know the pollen count and stay indoors when it is high.
—Close windows at night.
—Avoid outdoor activities from 5:00 A.M. to 10:00 A.M. when pollen is released. The pollen count declines as the day goes on.
—Keep car windows shut when driving.
—Do not mow the lawn during the grass pollen season, and stay away from freshly cut grass.
—Do not hang sheets or clothing out to dry. They collect pollen.

Herbal Remedies. Block or ease allergy symptoms with herbs. They work at the "mast-cell" level (located in your connective tissue). These "mast cells" release chemicals during inhalation to cause the allergic reaction. Herbs help prevent the "mast cells" from this release. Check the problem and herbal remedy:

General Ill Feeling: Drink one cup of an infusion of goldenrod tea. Repeat throughout the day.

Irritated Mucous Membranes. Drink one cup of a warm infusion of either of these herbal teas: hyssop, lavender, marjoram, thyme.

Itching Eyes. Apply cold compresses of witch hazel diluted in four parts boiled water to soothe your eyes.

Excess Mucus. Sip eyebright tea.

Eye Redness. Drink hot mullein flower tea and also eyebright tea.

Beware of Stress. It can trigger an allergic response or worsen existing symptoms. Reschedule activities to keep stress under control. It can be devastating!

Salt Water Rinse. Rinsing your nasal passages with ordinary salt water can be very soothing. Mix ¼ teaspoon salt in one cup of warm water. Then squirt the solution into your nose with a syringe.

HEADACHE

Symptoms

Describing a headache is simple—a pain in the head from the brow up. The ache ranges from a passing hurt to a full-blown eruption of agony. Several areas of your head can hurt, including a network of nerves that extend over your scalp, and certain nerves in your face, mouth, and throat. Also sensitive to pain, because they contain delicate nerve fibers, are the muscles of your head and blood vessels found along the surface and at the base of your brain. The bones of your skull and the tissues of your brain itself, however, never hurt, because they lack pain-sensitive nerve fibers. There are different causes and types of headaches, each with its natural remedy. Look for these reasons . . . and helps . . .

Natural Remedies

Here is a list of factors that may trigger headaches and suggestions on how to relieve them speedily.

1. *Sudden Salt Overload.* You may be sensitive to too much salt (sodium chloride). Heavily salted nuts or chips, especially on an empty stomach, can trigger a headache. Eliminate salty snacks, salt in food of any sort, and you may eliminate headaches.

2. *Caffeine Withdrawal Headache.* If you drink a lot of coffee, tea or soft drinks and suddenly kick the habit, you can react with headaches that may last for three to six hours. Caffeine constricts blood vessels; a sudden withdrawal causes the vessels to dilate, giving you a rebound headache. Taper off caffeine products gradually to avoid this type of headache.

3. *Hot Dog Headache Syndrome.* Hot dogs and sausages contain nitrite and nitrate preservatives that dilate blood vessels in the head to bring on headaches. Avoid processed meats and avoid this type of headache.

4. *Ice Cream Headache.* The sudden cooling of the roof of your mouth and throat overactivate nerves in that region to bring on a sudden headache. Go easy on ice-cold foods . . . or at least eat ice cream slowly, a little at a time.

5. *Cheese.* It causes more headaches than you suspect. Cheese contains tyramine, a breakdown product from the fermentation process in which it is manufactured. Yellow cheese has more tyramine than white cheese. The tyramine in cheese is one reason for the so-called "pizza headache." Limit cheese intake . . . and see if you can have pizza without the cheese.

6. *Hunger Headache.* If your blood sugar drops, you develop hypoglycemia and the symptom of a headache. This happens if you go without food for a long time. The remedy is to eat small meals throughout the day. A high protein snack made out of peas, beans, nuts, seeds, lean meat, and fish will help balance your blood sugar and avoid this type of headache.

7. *Cleaning Fluids Headache.* Irritating fumes from cleaning products—laundry soap, detergent, bleaches, etc.,—could bring on headaches. Use them in well-ventilated areas and try not to breathe in too deeply when in their presence.

8. *Alcohol Distress.* Alcohol is a vasodilator that opens up blood vessels, but chemicals in liquor joins with the alcohol to trigger headaches. The more costly liquor contains additives known as fusel oil and tailings, which provide flavor, but they are also "amines," which are powerful migraine or severe headache-producers. If you want to avoid headaches and improve your general health, avoid alcohol.

Natural "Aspirin." You are under stress, worry a lot, have endured some harrowing experiences . . . and develop a headache. Want relief? Concerned about the side effects of aspirin? Reach for a natural "aspirin" made from herbs. *Willow bark.* It was from this herb that the pain killers were first made before chemicals were used to create aspirin. *Willow bark,* available at your herbal pharmacist or health store, works by soothing your pain . . . yet it is natural and will not have the side effects of chemicalized aspirin.

Blame it on stress, not to mention erratic eating habits, with salty foods, Edward O'L. was plagued with recurring headaches that gripped him in a neck vise, causing excruciating and pounding pain. He took aspirin, but it caused ringing in his ears (he did not want any more head pain!) and internal bleeding. Was he doomed to stubborn headaches with their throbbing hurt? He might have been until a herbal pharmacist recommended he take a willow bark tablet as a substitute for aspirin. Edward O'L. tried it . . . and was almost immediately soothed . . . the pounding eased, and he felt welcome relief within thirty minutes. He eases up on his stress, avoids salty food to further protect against headaches, but with willow bark available, he is able to turn off "stubborn" headaches without the need for drugs.

HEARTBURN

Symptoms

Heartburn is usually a burning chest pain located behind the breast bone. Often there is a sensation of food coming back into the mouth, accompanied by an acid or bitter taste. Typically heartburn occurs after meals and is a common source of complaints of indigestion. Usually the burning-type chest pain lasts for many minutes—sometimes as long as two hours—and often is worse when you lie flat or bend over. Its full name is *gastroesophageal reflux*, but it is called heartburn because of the area in the body in which the burning sensation is felt. The condition is principally caused by the backup, or reflux, of acidic stomach contents into the esophagus (tube leading from the throat to the stomach). While generally not life-threatening, its unpleasant symptoms can be enervating and extremely discomforting.

Why Does It Happen? At the point where the esophagus joins the stomach, the esophagus is kept closed by a specialized muscle called the lower esophageal sphincter (LES). This is important, as the pressure in the stomach is normally higher than that in the esophagus. The muscle of the LES relaxes after swallowing to allow passage of food into the stomach, but then quickly closes again. *Problem*: Backwash of stomach contents into the esophagus, commonly called reflux, occurs when the LES muscle is very weak or, more commonly, when it inappropriately relaxes. The reflux tends to be worse after big meals and when you lie down at night.

Natural Remedies

There are specific steps to prevent heartburn that call for changes in your lifestyle. Donald O. Castell, M.D., Chief of the Gastroenterology Division at Wake Forest University's Bowman-Gray School of Medicine, in Winston Salem, N.C., offers these steps to put out the fire:

1. Watch your weight. Lose excess poundage. The pressure of extra weight can cause heartburn to occur more often.
2. Avoid wearing clothing that is too tight around stomach or waist.
3. Do not eat too fast. Take small mouthfuls and chew your food thoroughly.
4. Avoid bending forward, stooping and lifting heavy objects.
5. Sleep with the head of your bed elevated about six inches (perhaps by placing wooden blocks or bricks under the legs at the head of the bed.)
6. Keep a relaxed attitude in all your daily activities.
7. Cigarette smoking has been shown to decrease LES pressure dramatically, thus giving up the habit may help avoid heartburn.
8. Avoid talking while chewing or chewing with your mouth open since you might swallow too much air during the process.
9. All of us have foods that upset our digestive system. The hot peppers that another family member likes may be trouble for you. Find out which foods upset you and avoid them. Most are troubled by red wine, coffee, fried foods, spicy foods, chocolate. Again . . . if it upsets you, avoid it.
10. Eat at least two to three hours before lying down. Do **not** use extra pillows under your head, since they may only worsen the problem. If your body bends at the waist, you may be pushing the stomach contents upward—just what you do not want to do!

Food Program Prescribed. Dr. Castell suggests, "The ideal diet for the heartburn sufferer is high in protein and low in fat. I would recommend foods such as broiled (or baked) beef, chicken and fish; also skim milk and milk products. Other foods include potatoes, corn, apples, bananas, water, apple juice, baked cakes, soups (without garlic or onion), ice cream and some candies." Also, "An important solution to heartburn is prevention and that requires for you to be aware of your individual sensitivities and eat accordingly."[71]

Natural Antacids. To help neutralize stomach acids, herbal remedies produce a thick, foaming layer on top of stomach contents. This foam "raft" helps prevent the stomach contents from refluxing up into the esophagus and causing heartburn. These herbs neutralize the refluxed stomach contents before it has a chance to touch the lining of the esophagus. Put out the fire with these herbs:

Bitters. Available as capsules or liquid from your herbalist. Try goldenseal, gentian root or wormwood. A small amount before you eat can prevent heartburn.

Gingerroot. Calms your nerves and also helps to "soak up" the acid. Take two capsules right after you eat to buffer any attack.

Heartburn should not be ignored. If left untreated, chronic heartburn can lead to more serious medical problems. The constant backflow of acid can cause ulcers in the esophagus because its delicate tissues are vulnerable to injury by stomach acid and bile. This can lead to scarring of the esophagus and eventual narrowing.

HEMORRHOIDS

Symptoms

Hemorrhoids are simply varicose veins—enlarged, bulging veins—located in and around the rectum and anus. Also known as piles, they do not always cause pain or bleeding. Problems can occur when these veins become swollen because pressure is raised in them. Increased pressure may result from straining to move your bowels, from sitting too long on the toilet, or from other factors, such as pregnancy, obesity, or liver disease. There are two basic types of hemorrhoids: (1) *internal hemorrhoids* occur higher up in the anal canal, out of sight; irritation, resulting from constipation and straining can cause them to bleed. (2) *External hemorrhoids* form just outside the rectal canal in the anal lining and are visible. They are basically skin-covered veins that have ballooned and appear blue. When inflamed, they become red and tender. There may be pain and swelling, burning, and itching of the overlying skin. If you see blood in the stool or on the toilet tissue, check with your doctor to rule out more serious conditions.

Natural Remedies

You can follow simple programs that not only will lessen your chances of getting hemorrhoids but will keep them from getting more serious.

Boost Fiber Intake. Grandma was right in insisting you eat your roughage or dietary fiber. This plant food is not broken down during digestion but creates bulky and soft stool. To feed more fiber to your digestive system, try these tasty treats:

- Bran foods, such as bran cereals, whole wheat bread, and other whole-grain baked goods.
- Green leafy vegetables, such as celery, lettuce.
- Vegetables such as turnips, cabbage and carrots.
- Fresh fruits, especially plums, apricots, apples.
- Stewed or canned fruits, such as prunes or figs.
- Fruit juices—orange juice, prune, or fig juice. (All fruit juices add liquid and help avoid constipation.)
- Important foods are peas, beans, nuts, and fruits with the peel.

More Daily Exercise. Fitness gives better tone to the supporting muscles of the anorectal area as well as to the abdomen. Additionally, by increasing the movement of food through your body, exercise helps avoid constipation.

Proper Hygiene. This means carefully cleansing and removing irritation-causing matter that may cause pain, swelling, and itching. Washing, rinsing, and drying should be done gently to protect the sensitive tissue.

Drink Lots of Liquids. Your digestive system works best if you drink a minimum of six large glasses of liquids daily—fruit or vegetable juice, water, herbal tea. Do this without fail!

Establish Regularity. Train your bowel to maintain a routine. Whether or not you feel the need, go to the bathroom at the same time every day—especially after a meal, when your digestive process is naturally stimulated. Answer Nature's call promptly. The longer the wastes remain in your lower bowel, the drier and harder they become. Do **not** strain during bowel movements, since this aggravates hemorrhoids. If you haven't moved your bowels within a few minutes, get up and try again later. CAREFUL: Blood can accumulate in the rectal area and lead to hemorrhoids if you strain for long periods. *Note:* Don't be concerned if you only move your bowels every other day or have two or more movements a day. Every person is different. In most cases, what is "normal" is what is regular for you.

Warm Sitz Baths. Sitting on a folded bath towel in a tub with a few inches of warm—not hot—water for 15 minutes, three or four times a day, helps ease pain by relaxing muscles and soothing the anal area.

Comfort Cushions. Donut-shaped cushions can help to relieve pressure. They may be useful if you sit for long periods.

Cold Packs. If you know you are having pain from hemorrhoids, you might try putting cold packs on your anus, followed by a sitz bath, three or four times a day. To protect against irritation, cleanse the area carefully and apply petroleum jelly to the area.

Easy Does It. Avoid heavy lifting and extended bouts of sitting or standing because these practices tend to increase pressure on the rectum and worsen hemorrhoids. Limit sitting or standing periods to no more than 30 minutes at a time. Break up your day with frequent walks or rest periods with your legs raised.

Witch Hazel Remedy. For external hemorrhoids, especially if there is bleeding, dip a cotton ball in witch hazel and apply to the rectum area. Barbers have long used witch hazel if they cut you because it helps the blood vessels shrink down.

Cold Witch Hazel. Cool off the pain of hemorrhoids by putting a bottle of witch hazel in a bucket of ice. Let it become very cold, as you would champagne. Then soak a cotton ball in some iced witch hazel and apply to your hemorrhoids for as long as it feels cold. Then repeat several more times.

HEPATITIS

Symptoms

Hepatitis means inflammation (swelling and tenderness) of the liver. It is caused by several viruses that mainly attack the liver. It may also be caused by non-viral substances such as alcohol, chemicals, and drugs. There are two different types:

Hepatitis A. Spread through contaminated water and food; excreted in the stools. Food handlers, at home or in restaurant kitchens, should brush fingernails daily and wash their hands, especially after use of the toilet, to protect against transferring any virus in their intestinal and urinary tracts. Symptoms, which may be mild or severe, include nausea, fatigue, fever, abdominal discomfort, darkening of the urine, loss of appetite, jaundice (yellowing of eyes and skin). **DANGER:** If you travel to certain areas where food and water supplies may be contaminated, you are cautioned to drink only bottled, boiled, or otherwise effectively treated water. Avoid ice. Accept only cooked food and fruits that have been thoroughly washed and then peeled by the person who is going to eat them.

Hepatitis B. This is a liver disease caused by a virus carried in the blood, saliva, semen, and other body fluids of an infected person. It is acquired from transfusions or other blood products. It can be transmitted through minute cuts or abrasions, or by such simple acts as kissing, tooth brushing, ear piercing, tattooing, having dental work, or during sexual contact. Symptoms may include tiredness, poor appetite, fever, vomiting, joint pain, hives, rash or jaundice. The liver often becomes tender and enlarged. Doctors prescribe bed rest for those with Hepatitis B. Most people recover, but some become long-term carriers of the virus, and can spread it to others through sex and needle sharing.

Natural Remedies

Healing hepatitis calls for rest, a well-balanced, nutritious diet, and monitoring by a health practitioner. To prevent the spread of the infection, never touch any contaminated bowel movements. Use a disinfectant to clean the toilet. It is vital for you to wash your hands frequently.

Avoid irritating an already irritated liver by keeping away from alcohol and certain drugs which worsen the situation. These include tranquilizers, certain tetracyclines, antibiotics, antidepressants, high-dosage acetaminophens . . . or aspirin products. Discuss their use with your health practitioner.

Nutritional Healers. Nourish your liver with adequate amounts of vitamin A (fish liver oils, carrots, cantaloupe, peaches, squash, tomatoes, green and yellow fruits), vitamin B_6 (whole grain products, brewer's yeast, bananas, green leafy vegetables, wheat germ, pecans), vitamin B_{12} (liver, kidney, muscle meats—but these are also high in cholesterol and fat, so be cautious).

Your basic food program should be low-fat, high-fiber of minimally processed foods. If necessary, take a multiple vitamin-mineral supplement that provides no more than 300 percent of the RDA for all nutrients.

HERPES

Symptoms

Herpes—a name derived from the Greek for "to creep or crawl"—is a chronic, recurring, often very painful disease caused by the herpes simplex virus. People can be infected, yet have no symptoms; such people are carriers who can spread the disease to other, more susceptible people. It produces groups of blister-like sores about two to 14 days after infection. Sometimes a fever is present. The sores will break open and become painful, especially if they come in contact with urine. Even though the herpes sores may disappear, the virus is still present and the sores can return without warning. Spread through sexual contact is most likely to occur when sores are present. *Note*: Cold sores are also a form of herpes. People with sores on the mouth or lips should refrain from intimacies, since this may transfer the virus to the partner. The most prevalent forms are:

1. *Herpes simplex, type 1 (HSV-1)*. This is the common cold sore or fever blister, which cause the sores on the lips and mouth. If the eyes are affected, this is known as herpes keratitis. Wearers of contact lenses are especially susceptible to this ailment.

2. *Herpes simplex, type 2 (HSV-2)*. This is the common genital herpes. Sores appear on or around the sexual organs. These sores may itch, burn or be quite painful. They may be accompanied by swollen glands, general muscle aches, and fever.

What Triggers a Recurrence? Remember that both oral and genital herpes can recur, usually near the site of the initial infection. Herpes infections have different patterns in different people. Basically, any one or any combination of the following factors may sometimes—not always—induce an outbreak: surgery, illness, stress, fatigue, skin irritation (such as sunburn), diet, menstruation, or vigorous sexual intercourse.

Natural Remedies

During an outbreak, keep the infected area as clean and dry as possible. Some doctors recommend three warm showers per day in order to cleanse the infected area. Afterwards, towel dry gently or dry the area with a hair dryer on low or cool setting. Avoid tight-fitting undergarments.

Vitamin C. Some have found that doses of about 4,000 units daily help inactive the virus. Vitamin C also stimulates the immune system to resist the infection and minimize its symptoms.

Lysine. An amino acid that may help control the pain. In some reported tests, potencies ranging from 312 to 1,200 milligrams a day was found to be useful. Lysine also has an antagonistic effect on the substances that cause the reproduction of the herpes virus.

How to Relieve Itch. Tannic acid found in black teas relieves itching and some pain. Apply by placing a wet tea bag against the lesions. Cold milk compresses also reduce the itching and pain of lesions. Apply ice for a short time to lesions to ease discomfort. Lesions should be dried after ice is used.

Caring for Infected Area. Keep the area clean and dry. Warm water and soap will be adequate. Pat dry gently or blow dry with a hair dryer set on cool. CAREFUL: Moisture that occurs normally in the genital area can slow the healing process. Choose loose clothing that does not trap moisture. Cotton absorbs moisture—but synthetic materials such as nylon do not. Cotton underwear is preferable. Boxer shorts allow for more air circulation and drying than do snug fitting briefs. CAREFUL: Tight jeans that hold in moisture and chafe the genitals should be avoided, perhaps even between episodes.

Bathing, Drying, Powder. Drying agents such as epsom salts or Burrow's solution mixed in a warm bath may be beneficial. (Prolonged, frequent bathing may worsen the attack, so be careful not to overdo.) Cornstarch sprinkled on the genitals is an effective way of keeping the area drier. Almost any gentle non-irritating powder will also help with drying.

Personal Hygiene Tips. Be alert to the need for personal hygiene. Touching a sore and then touching some other part of your body can move the virus to a new location. This is especially true during the initial episode of the ailment. Fingers and eyes are particularly vulnerable, so exercise great caution and wash after touching the sores. These precautions should be followed for as long as the sores remain.

Don't ignore the need for proper nutrition, fitness and rest. Avoid stress, which not only weakens your immune system but could trigger an attack.

HIATAL HERNIA

Symptoms

In this ailment, a small portion of the stomach slips through an opening (hiatus) in the diaphragm, causing the stomach to "ride up" into the chest. The most frequent cause of hiatal hernia is an increased pressure in the abdominal cavity produced by coughing, vomiting, straining at the stool, or sudden physical exertion. A majority of people over 50 have hiatal hernias and, in most cases, they do not cause problems. There are indications that the condition runs in families, and those who are overweight.

Natural Remedies

A major problem is that the hiatus hernia is a pouch offshoot from the upper stomach/lower esophagus that catches acid-laden foods. This can be uncomfortable at mealtimes and for a while afterwards. To ease this distress, keep acid and spicy foods to a minimum.

Make some adjustments in your eating practices. *Problem*: You may try to swallow too much food too quickly and develop pockets of distension in your esophagus that cause discomfort whenever you eat. *Remedy*: Eat small bites. Eat slowly at the meal table. Chew thoroughly. Swallow small portions of food at a time.

After you eat, sit up in a chair. Avoid stooping, bending over or lying down because you do not want the food to "backwash" through the opening to cause distress.

Lose weight if you are too heavy. Follow a regular fitness program that improves your abdominal muscle tone and strengthens your diaphragm.

Loosen your garments. Restrictive clothing and tight belts increase stomach pressure and cause food in your stomach to back up.

Mealtime should be calm and pleasant. Stress is harmful because it affects the nerves that control the cardiac sphincter muscle and weakens the tension within it. Unrelieved stress at mealtimes will cause stomach contents to come back up into the upper part of your body.

Avoid smoking. It decreases lower esophagus sphincter (LES) pressure dramatically, which tends to dispatch the highly acidic contents of the stomach to back up. This backwash of stomach contents (reflux) irritates the lining of the esophagus, causing distress.

HYPERTENSION

Symptoms

Also known as high blood pressure, this ailment is an unstable or persistent elevation of blood pressure above the normal range. Uncontrolled, chronic high blood pressure strains the heart, damages arteries and creates a greater risk of heart attack, stroke and kidney problems. Called "the silent disease" for good reason—it has NO major symptoms! In some cases, hypertension may cause dizziness, headaches, fatigue, shortness of breath, nosebleeds and possible facial flushing. For the most part, this is a symptomless ailment.

To find out if you have high blood pressure, your doctor will probably take several readings using an instrument called a sphygmomanometer. The reading provides two numbers, the high or "systolic" number (when the heart beats) and a low or "diastolic" number (between heart beats).

How High Is Too High? The higher your diastolic blood pressure is, the greater your risk becomes of developing hypertension-related problems. Here is how doctors classify diastolic blood pressures, from least severe to most severe. The numbers are expressed in millimeters of mercury (mm Hg).

Classification	Diastolic Blood Pressure (mm Hg)
Normal	Less than 85
High Normal or Borderline	85–90
Mild	90–104
Moderately Severe	105–114
Severe	115–124

Best Reading. A blood pressure of 120/80 is believed to be the best, but there is no single blood pressure reading that is normal for everyone. Age, sex and overall health determine what is normal for you. And your blood pressure can be different at different times during the day. It is lowest when you are reading or sleeping. Physical or emotional stress can raise your pressure. Generally speaking, if your doctor tells you that you have hypertension, it almost always means your reading is above that of the "normal" 120/80. If it remains consistently above this level, it could, if not lowered, damage your heart, kidneys, eyes, and arteries.

Natural Remedies

To control your blood pressure, make easy adjustments in your living practices with these remedies.

Control Weight. Lose excess weight to help decrease the amount of excess blood pumped by your heart. This will also reduce pressure in your arteries. Above all, avoid overweight!

Limit Salt Intake. While the cause-and-effect relationship is unclear, it is known that salt sensitivity may cause a rise in blood pressure. Sodium or salt should be limited to help bring pressure under control. Read labels. Most packaged and processed foods contain salt and should thus be limited. This is especially important for older folks, who are more sensitive to salt.

Keep Yourself Fit. Regular aerobic exercise, the kind that raises your heart rate, if done continuously for 25 minutes or longer, five times a week, helps balance your blood pressure. A brisk 45-minute walk each day, or riding an exercise cycle for 45 minutes five times weekly can also be effective.

Stress-Tension. Reactions to stress, if you are stress-sensitive, can raise blood pressure. Follow stress soothing remedies, such as progressive muscle relaxation, yoga, meditation. A much calmer approach to life can help improve your blood pressure and general health.

Potassium. A helpful mineral tends to balance your blood pressure. A modest amount—as in two large bananas a day—is all you need. Bananas will also establish a natural diuretic effect to help clear salt out of your body.

What Do You Drink? Alcohol in moderate amounts is probably harmless but having more than two drinks a day may elevate blood pressure. Caffeine-containing drinks, such as coffee, tea, or colas, increase the rate at which your heart beats and thus may push your blood pressure higher. It is best to limit their intake.

Smoking Is Dangerous. Chemicals in tobacco can tighten your arteries, raising your pressure. There are additional dangers to heart and lungs. Smoking should be eliminated.

Garlic Helps Control Blood Pressure. In many reported tests, garlic has been shown to have a dilating effect on the blood vessels, helping to effectively reduce blood pressure. Several cloves of raw garlic daily as part of a salad may well be the best natural medicine to control your blood pressure.

Noise Raises Blood Pressure. Noise is a form of stress, which can raise blood pressure and circulatory disorders. It may come from alarm clocks jangling, loud work-place noises, blaring hi-fi stereo sets, yelling, ear-hurting radios or televisions . . . noise is hurtful and should be kept to a minimum. Shut out disturbing noises, and you may well help control blood pressure . . . not to mention other health benefits.

Magnesium: Important but Overlooked. The "neglected" mineral, magnesium should be considered as an important pressure-balancing element. It is known that magnesium influences how the heart and blood vessels contract and relax. DANGER: A deficiency of magnesium will cause artery walls to go into spasm and the heartbeat to become irregular. *Remedy*: With magnesium, the artery walls dilate (relax) and the heartbeat returns to normal. *Note*: Constriction and spasms of the arteries are associated with hypertension; it is magnesium that promotes dilation of the arteries, increases the size of the lumen (internal space such as blood vessel), reduces resistance to blood flow and helps lower blood pressure. Magnesium is available in whole grain foods, dry beans and peas, dark green vegetables, soy products, and also as a supplement.

Hypertension is a multifaceted ailment, and it is wise to consider a holistic or total body approach involving both emotional and physical components to help bring it under control.

HYPOGLYCEMIA

Symptoms

Also known as low blood sugar, this ailment often is accompanied by sweating, shakiness, trembling, anxiety, fast heart action, headache, hunger sensations, feelings of weakness and, occasionally, seizures, fainting episodes, and unconsciousness. In *reactive hypoglycemia*, the symptoms are more severe and are noticeable after a high carbohydrate meal. Large amounts of sugars and starches cause an overload as your body converts them to glucose. The reaction consists of your body producing too much insulin to metabolize the glucose, leading to low blood sugar and accompanying symptoms.

Natural Remedies

High sugar intake can upset your hormones and result in low blood sugar. To correct any imbalance, start with these basic natural remedies:

1. Eat small, frequent meals. When your blood glucose level begins to drop, a new meal offers an additional supply of carbohydrates to maintain good levels of blood glucose.

2. Either minimize or avoid alcohol, caffeine, and tobacco because they play havoc with a vengeance upon your blood sugar levels.

3. Exercise at least five times weekly for at least 45 minutes per session. Exercise boosts blood sugar regulation and the receptivity of your cells to insulin.

A Doctor's Plan for Better Energy. Holly Atkinson, M.D., author of *Women and Fatigue*, offers a set of natural remedies to protect against fatigue-causing hypoglycemia:

1 Make complex carbohydrates—starchy foods such as potatoes, pasta, bread, cereals, grains, peas and beans, and related foods— the mainstay of any meal. The best carbohydrates are unrefined and minimally processed; for example, whole wheat bread, brown rice and a baked potato. Carbohydrates are your body's preferred fuel. Without them, your body is forced to burn fats and protein (including muscles and organs) for energy, which causes the formation of fatigue-inducing toxic substances.

2. Avoid simple carbohydrates—the sugars, sweet snacks, and the like. Sugar provides a false and short-lived pick-me-up; within an hour or so, you are let down lower than before. If you crave a sweet treat after or between meals, choose naturally sweet and nutritious fruits, both fresh and dried.

3. Eat enough protein but not too much. Most folks consume two or more times the daily protein requirement. The average woman needs only 40 to 50 grams of protein a day. Three ounces of flounder, two cups of spaghetti and one cup of skim milk would supply 50 grams of protein. Excessive protein can result in a build-up of toxic wastes and put stress on the kidneys.

4. Design meals to maximize energy when it is needed most. Protein is a wake-up food that should be prominent at breakfast and lunch. At suppertime, a high-carbohydrate meal with little or no protein can be relaxing. **TIP:** It is better to eat several small

meals throughout the day than one or two large ones, which may cause sleepiness and sluggishness.

5. Don't skip meals or go on fasts. Hunger causes blood sugar levels to fall, and the likely consequence is feeling tired and irritable. Similarly, the binge-purge eating scheme used by people with bulimia to control weight is seriously energy-depleting.

6. Don't rely on caffeine as a pick-me-up. Caffeine is an addictive drug, and a dependent person is likely to feel especially tired between doses. A short catnap is a far better solution for midday sleepiness.[72]

Had Your Chromium Today? A little-known trace mineral, chromium is helpful to those with reactive hypoglycemia. It tends to stabilize the flow of insulin. CAREFUL: If you are diabetic, discuss chromium use with your practitioner. Otherwise, it is available in whole grains, and as a supplement.

CASE HISTORY—*Constant Fatigue, Emotional Upsets, Temperament Threaten Career Woman's Hard-Earned Promotion*

With her promotion came many new challenges and responsibilities that Barbara M. welcomed with ambition. She had to put in extra hours, with more pressure, in the marketing firm, which had her earmarked for a position as a member of the board of directors. In the midst of it all, she had bouts of fatigue, emotional collapses, and sharp temper. She could not follow a sensible food program and overloaded on convenience or snack foods that were almost all concentrated sugar. She had trouble with her vision, developed tremors, found it difficult to participate in vital business meetings. Barbara M. was on the verge of being fired if she did not correct her behavior. What was wrong?

An endocrinologist confirmed her hypoglycemia. He immediately told her to avoid refined carbohydrates and to eat more complex carbohydrates, such as whole grain pasta, beans, brown rice, fresh vegetables. These would take longer to be digested and would stabilize her blood glucose levels. Only moderate amounts of insulin would be produced. He recommended that she eat only small amounts of protein; that she drink less coffee, until it was eliminated—no caffeine from soft drinks or chocolate; and that she eat smaller meals, spaced throughout the day. Barbara M. recovered almost immediately. She became healthfully energetic. No more emotional tempers. Her vision improved. She had better cognitive (thought) control. She was in charge of herself! Her endocrinologist prescribed a small portion of daily protein with the complex carbohydrates to get her back to normal. In four weeks, Barbara M. was a happy and healthy career woman . . . and anticipated being voted as a member of the board of directors. She had controlled her blood sugar . . . and could now control her future!

HYPOTHERMIA

Symptoms

Take the person's temperature. If it is below 96°F (35.5°C), it may well be hypothermia. Other symptoms to look for include confusion, disorientation, drowsiness, slurred speech, shallow and very slow breathing, weak pulse, poor muscle coordination, uncontrollable shivering. In severe cases, body temperatures can drop below 84°F and muscle become rigid, extremities are purple, and loss of consciousness may occur. The elderly are especially vulnerable because of reduced resistance to and ability to recover from stresses, such as prolonged exposure to cold.

Natural Remedies

Follow these protective steps.

Clothing. Dress warmly in cold weather. Clothing is a good insulator especially when layered. Down or natural materials, such as cotton and wool, are the best insulators. Wearing a hat substantially reduces heat loss. Keep dry. Wet clothing is twenty times less effective than dry clothing.

Medications. Some may increase risk of accidental hypothermia. Such drugs include chlorpromazine and related medications given to treat anxiety depression and nausea. Some over-the-counter cold remedies may even make you more vulnerable. Discuss with your physician how your medication affects body heat.

Avoid Alcohol. It severely lowers the body's ability to retain heat. Alcohol dilates peripheral blood vessels and thus counters the body's mechanism for conserving heat.

When You Sleep. Have enough warm blankets. Socks and a nightcap, and even thermal underwear, help keep you warm while sleeping. **TIP:**

Use flannel sheets placed above a sheepskin or wool mattress cover for super-warmth. **Also:** use several light-weight blankets rather than one heavy blanket when sleeping.

If You Must Go Outside. Dress warmly in loose-fitting, layered, lightweight wool clothing. Outer garments should be tightly woven and water repellant. Wear a wool hat because your body loses between one-half and three-quarters of its heat through your head. Protect your face, and cover your mouth to protect your lungs from very cold air. Wear mittens instead of gloves—they allow your fingers to move freely in contact with one another and will keep your hands much warmer.

Quick Helps for Hypothermia Victim. Quickly do the following:

- Remove wet clothing and, if possible, get the person into a warm bed to prevent further heat loss.
- A person who is conscious and not coughing or vomiting can be given warm drinks—**not** alcohol, sedatives, tranquilizers or pain relievers. They only slow down body processes even more. Otherwise, give nothing by mouth.
- Do **not** pile heavy layers on top of the person. Do **not** rub cold limbs in an effort to warm them. Keep the person quiet. Do not jostle, massage, or rub.

Seek Medical Assistance. Hypothermia does not go away by itself, so seek prompt medical assistance. Rewarming should be done slowly—usually from the inside out—by professionals. **DANGER:** Rapid rewarming dilates blood vessels near the skin, further lowering blood pressure and dispatching more cold blood to the body core.

Indoors? Warm Enough for You? Room temperatures below 70°F could be dangerous if you are not dressed warmly enough. If this happens, be sure to put on a hat. This sends more warm blood to your hands and feet. Use a warm scarf to cover your neck. If you live alone, you may neglect yourself and risk extended exposure to the cold. Take better care of yourself! Eat well-balanced, nutritious meals, to allow your body to produce its own heat efficiently, such as complex carbohydrates, soups, warm caffeine-free beverages. Keep yourself and your clothes dry. Change wet socks and all other wet clothing as quickly as possible to prevent loss of body heat. **DANGER:** Wet clothing loses all of its insulating value and evaporates heat rapidly.

❧ 1 ❧

IMMUNE SYSTEM

Symptoms

Every second of every day, your body engages in a fight for its life. It is constantly battling assaults by enemies ranging from infectious organisms to harmful chemicals to cancerous cells. If your body is healthy, it has the means with which to win these battles—namely, the white blood cells and molecules of your immune system. This "inner fortress" gathers an abundance of phagocytes, neutrophils, macrophages, lymphocytes to "disarm" the hordes of threatening bacteria and viruses.

Your thymus (an organ in your chest) dispatches T-cells to rid your body of diseased or abnormal cells. Symptoms may be a cold, premature aging, organ illness, cancer, infection of any sort. Your immune system rises to the occasion to overcome the invaders, using antibodies for inner detoxification. A strong and healthy immune system is your key to youthful health and freedom from illness.

Natural Remedies

Nutrition plays a major role in the health and functioning of your immune system. All organs, cells and chemicals in the immune system are directly affected by your nutritional status. Even marginal deficiencies of one or more nutrients can have pronounced effects on immunocompetence. The important immune-boosting nutrients include:

Vitamin A or beta-carotene. Involved in cell growth and differentiation and also reproduction. This vitamin functions as a quencher of free radicals—a valuable function because free radicals are "destroyed" in the biochemistry of your body, weakening your immune system, bringing on cellular deterioration and aging. Beta-carotene is a thirsty sponge that soaks up the dangerous free radicals that destroy cells.

Free radicals are a class of highly corrosive, oxidizing molecules which are fragmented and unstabled. They have unattached electrons which cause them to attack cells in order to complete themselves. These are toxic chemical substances that attack your body's cells. They contribute to the development of heart disease, cancer, stroke, arthritis, diabetes and other age-associated disorders chiefly because they weaken the cell's ability to repair itself. Where do they come from? They are introduced into your body through improper diet, tobacco, alcohol, stress, polluted air, background radiation, and even your body's own natural processes. Beta-carotene acts as a bodyguard for your immune system, repels foreign invaders, stimulates your resistance to many ailments involving cellular destruction.

Vitamin C. Stimulates your immune system to attack and detoxify abnormal cells. It is a free radical cleanser, mopping up free radicals, to prevent destruction of your Deoxyribonucleic acid, or DNA (genetic code). It is especially powerful in producing interferon, a potent disease-fighter in the body. This vitamin helps manufacture more T-cells, to form antibodies that will fight disease and, as a bonus, repair damaged tissues.

Vitamin E. A fat-soluble antioxidant in blood plasma, vitamin E helps sweep out waste materials and builds a stronger cellular fortress. It is "food" for your immune system. It bolsters the production of antibodies and protects against fungal and bacterial infections.

Zinc. This mineral is needed for new cell growth. Wound recovery calls for adequate quantities of zinc. The mineral also boosts production of immune "soldiers" that battle invading organisms. Zinc is also directly toxic to invading bacteria and viruses. Zinc invigorates your immune system, to help you resist common and uncommon ailments.

Selenium. This trace element protects prostacyclin (hormone-like substance) needed to promote immune power. Selenium acts as a shield for your body's "soldiers," as they douse the invading organisms with lethal free radicals. This mineral is involved in killing off dangerous bacteria and viruses without upsetting your immune system. With adequate selenium, your immune system is able to produce sufficient antibodies to repel invading foreign viruses. *Unique Combination.* Selenium with vitamin E combine to activate the production of an anti-aging enzyme called *glutathione peroxidase* (GSH). This enzyme is a dynamic inner cleanser. It wipes out renegade cells and dangerous free radicals and promotes healing from within via an invigorated immune system.

Build a Stronger Immune System with Nutrition. These nutrients form the foundation for a stronger immune system. Daily intake from foods and supplements will help strengthen your "inner fortress" to repel microorganisms and also overcome those that penetrate your body, so that you will have a younger and healthier lifestyle.

INCONTINENCE

Symptoms

Loss of bladder control affects up to 11 million people. Its causes range from a complication of constipation to serious neuromuscular disease. At least one in ten persons aged 65 or older has an incontinence problem, ranging from slight losses of urine to disability, or even immobility from more frequent wetting. Stress incontinence (not to be confused with anxiety and psychological stress) describes the leakage of urine during exercise, coughing, sneezing, laughing, and other body movement that puts pressure on the bladder. It occurs when the pelvic muscles are too relaxed to hold the bladder in position, or it can occur when the sphincter is damaged. Diabetes, pelvic trauma, lesions or injuries to the spinal cord can all cause loss of muscle tone. The most common obstructions are caused by enlargement of the prostate gland. Additionally, stroke, senile dementia, Alzheimer's disease and multiple sclerosis can all cause uninhibited incontinence. Incontinence may be a symptom—perhaps the first and only symptom—of a urinary tract infection. It may also occur in otherwise normal elderly persons.

Natural Remedies

Various programs are available to help control the urge to void. One or more may be useful.

Behavioral Management. Biofeedback is one method that is based on the recognition that when you feel some rectal distension, you can be trained to tighten the contractions of your external anal sphincter. You thereby gain control over your bladder. Management techniques can be taught so you can consciously delay voiding.

Weight Reduction. Weight losses of as little as 5 to 10 percent of body weight can significantly reduce stress incontinence caused by excessive intra-abdominal pressure in obese individuals.

Pelvic Floor Exercises. E. Douglas Whitehead, M.D., Assistant Clinical Professor of Urology at Mount Sinai School of Medicine, in New York City, suggests these exercises, which are designed to strengthen the pelvic floor muscles, as well as a squeezing action that will help hold back the flow of urine.

1. Sit or stand. Without tensing the muscles of your legs, buttocks or abdomen, imagine that you are trying to hold back a bowel movement by tightening the ring of muscle around your anus. Do this exercise only until you identify the back part of the pelvic floor.

2. When you are passing urine, try to stop the flow, then restart it. This will help you identify the front part of the pelvic floor. Now you are ready to do the major exercise that follows.

3. Working from back to front, tighten the muscles while counting to four slowly, then release them. You can do this exercise anywhere—sitting or standing, while watching TV or waiting for a bus. There is no need to interrupt your normal daily activity. Do not tighten your abdominal, thigh or buttock muscles, or cross your legs, in order to feel only the pelvic muscles. *Note:* Do this exercise for at least two minutes, three or more times daily (at least 100 repetitions).

4. Start and stop your stream five times each time you urinate. That is, start the flow of urine. Squeeze to hold back, let go to resume the flow. Hold back, let go, etc. Remember, do this every time you urinate. You probably will notice that you have much more control of the flow of urine in the morning than you do in the afternoon. That is because your muscles are not so tired.

"These exercises are fairly simple to learn and can be done any time. Once you've learned the feel of it, you can practice tightening and relaxing this muscle anywhere without anyone knowing you're doing it. Ask your doctor for assistance in learning how. It may take several months to see a real difference but the more you do it, the better the results," says Dr. Whitehead.[73]

Less Fluids-Empty Bladder. You may be drinking too many liquids. Keep a diary and write down exactly how many glasses of liquids you drink daily. Ease up . . . especially before bedtime. Do **not** drastically restrict fluid intake without your doctor's approval, lest you develop dehydration. Generally speaking, less is better.

Three Substances to Avoid. Keep away from

1. Alcohol because it is an uncontrollable diuretic and you don't need that!

2. Caffeine will also keep sending you to the bathroom. It is found in coffee, soft drinks, but also in commercial tea, chocolate, and many medications.

3. Grapefruit juice may have nutrients, but it also acts as a strong diuretic and is best avoided if you are incontinent.

Avoid Smoking. Nicotine acts as an abrasive to the surface of the bladder and irritates your elimination organs. CAREFUL: Smoker's cough is not only physically dangerous, but it triggers leakage!

Establish Regularity. Get into the habit of regular visits to the bathroom. Never . . . but never hold it in because of embarrassment while at the dinner table. You can develop infection along with overstretching of your bladder. CAREFUL: If you neglect the urge, your full bladder presses on your weak sphincter muscle and the least cough, laugh or sneeze will be embarrassing!

INDIGESTION

Symptoms

Also known as dyspepsia, this condition refers to painful, difficult, or disturbed digestion. You are said to have indigestion if you have several of a group of symptoms that might include nausea, regurgitation (backwash of stomach contents into the esophagus or mouth), vomiting, heartburn, prolonged upper abdominal fullness or bloating after a meal, stomach discomfort or pain, and early fullness. Often people say they have a "sick feeling in the stomach," or "nervous stomach," when they have dyspeptic symptoms. You may experience these symptoms after overeating or eating foods that disagree with you. Sometimes the symptoms accompany another condition, such as peptic ulcer disease, gallbladder problems, or gastritis. Symptoms may last for three to four days, sometimes longer. They may be severe and continuous, disrupting daily routines and causing absences from work.

Natural Remedies

William Y. Chey, M.D., Clinical Professor of Medicine at the University of Rochester School of Medicine, in Rochester, New York, tells us, "If your doctor has ruled out a specific illness causing your dyspepsia, your symptoms can probably be controlled if you take the following dietary precautions:

• Avoid greasy foods or solid foods containing meat.

- If you are lactose intolerant, eliminate milk and milk products.
- If your symptoms are severe, follow a liquid diet or eat soft foods in small amounts until your symptoms subside.

"It is well known that dyspepsia-like symptoms can accompany emotional upsets, although they may not be the most common cause or even the precipitating factor. Before emotional tension or distress can be named as the culprit causing dyspepsia, your doctor will conduct a careful medical evaluation to rule out other factors."[74]

Taking Care of Your Digestive System. Keep this system working at its best with these suggestions:

- Eat a well-balanced diet that includes a variety of fresh fruits, vegetables, and whole grain breads, cereals, and other grain products.
- Eat slowly. Whenever possible, try to relax for 30 minutes after each meal.
- Exercise regularly, at least 45 minutes a day.
- Avoid alcohol and caffeine.

How to Reduce Gas in Your Digestive Tract. Occasionally, gas collects in some portion of the digestive tract, a situation that can lead to pain or bloating. Why does it happen? Harris R. Clearfield, M.D., an expert on gastroenterology and Professor of Medicine at Hahnemann Medical College and Hospital of Philadelphia, Pennsylvania explains, "The most common source of gas is swallowed air. Each time you swallow, small amounts of air enter your stomach. There may be upper abdominal pressure and pain after eating." Dr. Clearfield offers these suggestions on reducing gas:

- Eat meals slowly and chew your food thoroughly.
- Check with a dentist to make sure dentures fit properly.
- Avoid chewing gum or sucking on hard candies.
- Eliminate carbonated beverages such as beer and soda from your diet.
- Avoid milk and milk products if you are lactose intolerant.
- Eat fewer gas-producing foods such as cauliflower, Brussels sprouts, bran, beans, broccoli, and cabbage.
- Try exercises such as situps to increase tone if abdominal distention is a problem.

- Always eat with your mouth closed.
- Do not drink out of bottles or cans; do not drink through a straw.
- Avoid foods that have a high air content such as beer, ice cream souffles, omelets, and whipped cream.[75]

INSECT BITES

Symptoms

A sting may cause itching, swelling, redness, rash, and varying degrees of pain. Insect stings are more than an annoyance. One of every 250 persons is highly allergic to insect attacks. Reactions can involve an entire limb or the whole body. Degrees of reaction are: 1) *Slight*—hives, itching, fatigue, anxiety feelings. 2) *Moderate*—swelling, tightness of chest, dizziness, abdominal cramps, nausea and/or vomiting may be present. 3) *Severe*—difficulty swallowing and breathing, weakness, confusion. 4) *Shock*—severe drop in blood pressure, difficulty breathing, swelling of face and lips.

While some individuals will react immediately to the sting, others may feel reaction several hours or even two weeks later.

Natural Remedies

It is possible to avoid the risk of insect stings by heeding some of the following suggestions, as offered by Jerome Z. Litt, M.D., dermatologist at Case Western Reserve University of Medicine, Cleveland, Ohio,

- Always wear shoes outside. Bare feet are the most vulnerable area for insect attacks. (Bees love clover, and yellow jackets live in the ground.)
- Avoid scented soaps, perfumes, colognes, hair sprays, and other scented products. These odors attract insects.
- Wear light-colored, smooth fabrics. Bright, flowery prints and dark, rough clothing attract insects as well.
- Avoid bright jewelry and other metal objects. Again, insects find these very alluring.
- If you come in contact with a stinging insect, avoid sudden and dramatic motions. Move away very slowly. Do not flap, wave or swat.
- Avoid touching insect nests.

• Keep house screens in good repair. Keep garbage cans covered at all times. Be especially alert after rain; pollen is scarce, and insects become more easily excited.

Quick Help For Stings. Dr. Litt explains that the treatment for most insect bites and stings is the same. "In the case of a bee sting, remove the barbed stinger and attached venom sac as quickly as possible, since the walls of the sac contract and continue to inject venom.

CAREFUL: "Never try to pull the stinger out or squeeze the area in which the stinger is embedded. This will break the venom sac, releasing more of the toxic or allergic substances and aggravating your symptoms. Instead, gently scrape the area with a knife blade or fingernail until the stinger and sac have been dislodged."

After you remove both stinger and venom sac, Dr. Litt suggests you follow these steps to treat the simple insect sting:

• Wash the area with soap and water.
• Use ice packs or cold compresses for 30 to 45 minutes to reduce the inflammation and swelling.
• Apply a paste made up of one teaspoonful of unseasoned meat tenderizer and water. This often results in prompt, lasting relief.
• For a few, localized insect bites, where there is redness, swelling and itching, the best immediate treatment is applying ice. An ice cube, held on the bite areas for five to ten minutes will usually give prompt relief from the pain, itching, and swelling.[76]

Treating a Sting. For bee, wasp, and hornet stings, remove the stinger. Then apply an alkali . . . ammonia water or bicarbonate of soda . . . at once to counteract the acid of the stinger's poison. Then apply witch hazel to the area.

Are You Allergic? You may go into shock! An ordinary bee sting may cause abnormal swelling, massive hives, wheezing and difficulty in breathing, diarrhea, a drop in blood pressure. Prompt attention by a physician is mandatory. For mild, local reactions, a cool compress or an ice bag are helpful. People who have severe allergies to bee stings can also wear protective nets when they are near bees—or run the risk of being stung. Anyone who has ever had a severe reaction to a bee sting (not just swelling and pain around the sting) in the past should seek medical help immediately, if stung. *Suggestion*: Stay indoors immediately after a rain when insects are especially active. Don't drink or eat outdoors. Delegate someone else to do gardening or outdoor work.

What About Heat? Ironically, heat can ease distress because it neutralizes a chemical that causes inflammation. TIP: Aim a hair dryer at your sting!

Aspirin Is Relieving. Moisten the sting. Rub an ordinary aspirin tablet into it. Ingredients in the aspirin neutralize hurtful inflammatory substances in the venom, to provide relief.

Give the Sting a Mud Remedy. Mix a small amount of water and clay soil until you have a mud paste. Apply to the sting. Cover with plastic wrap or gauze or a clean cloth. Let it remain until the mud dries. It helps take the heat out of the sting and protects against swelling and hurt.

Nutritional Remedy. Vitamin B_1 (thiamine) is said to create a natural insect repellent in human skin. Taking 50 milligrams per day may well help build your resistance to insect bites.

Don't Scratch! It may provide some relief, but it can lead to a secondary infection that may require internal antibiotic therapy. Use the natural remedies quickly to help calm down that itch. If it persists, consult with a dermatologist. It may not be a simple itch after all.

INSOMNIA

Symptoms

After a long, hard day you snuggle beneath the covers, exhausted, hoping to drift off into pleasant dreamland. You end up tossing and turning, your mind racing ahead. Your bedside alarm clock keeps ticking away. If only you could fall asleep. All too soon, it is time to get up for the next day. You feel exhausted after another battle with insomnia. An occasional sleepless night is no cause for alarm. It is usually a reaction to stress—personal, jet lag, change in routine, some anxiety. If insomnia becomes chronic, in which deep sleep is unattainable, it calls for corrective healing. Because sleep needs vary greatly, the term "insomnia" is defined as the perception of inadequate sleep, combined with impaired daytime performance. If you are tired, irritable, unable to function the next day, you need help for your insomnia.

Natural Remedies

Although sleep is a natural physiological reaction, it is basically *a learned behavior*. You can get yourself into a "sleep routine" with some basic guidelines:

Sleep Hygiene. Go to bed and get up at the same time each day, even on weekends. Use your bedroom only for sleep. Do not fight sleep but let sleepiness be a signal to go to bed!

Avoid Stimulants. Although alcohol can cause sleepiness, it seriously disturbs sleep, causing both fragmented sleep and early morning awakenings. Coffee, tea, colas, and other stimulants should also be avoided, especially in the evening. You may give up these stimulants entirely to enjoy better sleep.

Fitness-Relaxation. Light exercise performed regularly but not too close to bedtime will help your chances of enjoying deep sleep. Relaxation training will also be of use in helping you overcome sleep-onset difficulties.

Five Steps to Drift Off Into Dreamland. Peter Hauri, M.D., director of the Mayo Clinic Insomnia Program, tells us that for better snoozing, you may need to improve your sleeping habits. He suggests this basic five-step natural program:

1. Cut down on your sleeptime. If you need eight hours of sleep, then you should stay in bed eight hours, not ten. The longer you stay in bed, the shallower your sleep becomes. And your sleep is not as restorative.
2. Never try to sleep. The harder you try, the more likely you are to remain awake. Sleep can come only if you don't force it. Try engaging in some distractions: read, listen to quiet music. If you read, use adequate light but don't blast yourself with bright light.
3. Don't be afraid of insomnia. Don't let yourself get uptight if you can't get to sleep. You will still be able to function tomorrow.
4. Let rituals work for you. Listen to your favorite program, change into pajamas or gown, brush your teeth. You'll become more relaxed and comfortable as you do these things. Get yourself into this "sleep routine."
5. Give yourself time to wind down. You cannot expect to be at full speed at 11:00 P.M., and fall asleep at 11:05 P.M.

"Many insomniacs may not ever become champion Olympian sleepers," says Dr. Hauri, "but if they follow these simple steps, they'll sleep better."[77]

The Herb that Helps You Sleep . . . Naturally. Valerian root is an herb available in capsule form at most health stores. It has a reputation for helping you relax, almost like a natural sedative. Its ingredients soothe your nerves and give you a comfortable feeling, conducive to refreshing sleep. Noted herbalist, Michael A. Weiner, M.S., M.A., Ph.D., of San Rafael, California, author of *Weiner's Herbal*, explains, "In an age of anxiety, when tranquilizing agents reign supreme, it may be wise to reconsider the natural sedatives. Of the many plants employed to calm nervous patients, quiet hysteria or allay the fears of hypochondriacs, none seems to come forward with such recommendations as valerian root. It is a non-narcotic, perfectly safe herbal sedative and is highly recommended in anxiety states."[78]

Soothing Ways to Enjoy Sleep. Specialists with the Lenox Hill Hospital Sleepline, in New York City offer this set of guidelines for natural sleep. "Learn these four steps to natural, drug-free sleep for use whenever you have a sleep problem. Many people seem to have lost the ability to fall asleep naturally these days. However, learning to sleep can be enjoyable and soothing."

1. *Motionless Lying.* Find a comfortable position and try to lie as still as possible—no moving. For many people, motionless lying is adequate all by itself to get to sleep. If at first you want to move, try to overcome this restlessness and remain still. The urge to move will pass. If you move, you disturb your nervous system and start the wakefulness cycle again. So find a good position and remain as still as possible.

2. *Relax Your Muscles.* Become aware of your muscles, one by one, by tensing and then releasing the tension. Start with the big toe on your left foot—tense, then release, and be aware of the relaxation. Then repeat with your next toe, and your third, fourth and fifth. Repeat with your right toes, tense and release 1, 2, 3, 4, 5. Then your left foot and right. Repeat the tension and release to relaxation, first on the left, then the right, with your calf and thigh, your fingers, hands, arms, and shoulders. Then tense and release your stomach muscles and your neck. Be aware of the relaxation and the feeling of heaviness that enters your body. Tense and release your facial muscles, your lips and your brow. Be aware of the relaxation. Throughout the exercise, continue your motionless lying.

3. *Slow Your Breathing.* As you become more relaxed, be aware of your breathing and let it go a little slower. Take a deep breath, let it out slowly, and swallow very comfortable. Relax and allow your breathing to come more slowly.

4. *Prepare For Dreaming.* Review the events of your day. Let a mental tape run backwards in your head. As you see each event, either dwell on it, or skip to the next event, as you wish. It is unimportant whether your eyes are open or closed. Let your mind relax as it passes backwards over the events of the day. Your mind will feel refreshed as it prepares to go to sleep. Let your mind wander, to comforts, to enjoyments, and see them in mental pictures as you prepare for dreaming. Enjoy that good, drifting, dreaming feeling as sleep begins to near. Let go and relax. You will soon be asleep.

The Lenox Hill Hospital sleep specialists caution, "Avoid the use of chemicals such as sleeping pills, tranquilizers or alcohol. Although they may help at first, long term use can interfere with normal sleep patterns. **TIP:** If you want a beverage before bed, have a glass of warm milk, which contains the amino acid L-tryptophan, a natural tranquilizer."[79]

Nature's Sleeping Pill. Foods containing the amino acid L-tryptophan may well work as an all-natural sleeping pill. These include milk, tuna fish, cottage cheese, soybeans, cashews, chicken, turkey, and sardines (with bones). Include these "sandman snacks" as part of your regular food program to help yourself enjoy soothing sleep . . . naturally.

Hints, Tips, Suggestions. Wear eyeshades to screen out undesirable light. Earplugs help block out excessive noise, especially if you live near a busy intersection. Wear night clothing that is neither too tight nor too loose. Your bedsheets should be smooth. Find your personal sleep pattern. Go to sleep at the same time every night. Get up at the same time every morning. Natural fibers—silk, linen, wool, and cotton—are your best choices for bedding, to avoid static electricity that comes from rubbing against synthetic fibers. During sleep, you breathe approximately 30 barrels of air; keep your windows open, if only a crack. The best sleep temperature is between 60°F and 64°F. Lower temperatures will make you require more sleep to feel rested; higher temperatures will cause you to be restless during sleep. If the temperature is higher than 70°F, you may not sleep long enough.

IRRITABLE BOWEL SYNDROME

Symptoms

Also known as IBS, spastic colon, mucous colitis, this syndrome is a functional disorder that results in changes in the pattern of colon movements. Common symptoms include gas, bloating, abdominal pain, diarrhea or constipation, or the cyclical occurrence of both. Most people with IBS have episodes of lower abdominal pain and constipation sometimes followed by diarrhea. This ailment may be caused by emotional conflict or stress, or improper nutrition which react upon the colon.

Natural Remedies

In people who have IBS, the muscle of the lower portion of the colon contracts abnormally to be felt as a spasm or crampy pain. To ease this situation, be good to your colon by following these basic guidelines:

Avoid Stress. It can trigger painful spasms. Your nervous system influences your colon, and if you are "up tight" or "all wound up," your colon reacts with painful spasms.

Reduce Fat Intake. Sidney Cohen, M.D., Professor of Medicine at the University of Pennsylvania, and an expert on IBS, tells us, "Eating causes contractions of the colon. In people with IBS, the exaggerated reflex can lead to cramps and sometimes diarrhea. The strength of the response is directly related to the number of calories in a meal, especially the amount of fat in that meal. Fat in any form (animal or vegetable) is the strongest stimulus of colonic contractions after a meal. Fat is primarily found in meats, especially bacon and sausage; poultry skin, dairy products including milk, cream, cheese and butter; vegetable oils; margarines; shortenings; non-dairy whipped toppings." Dr. Cohen notes that this fat will stimulate colonic spasm if you have IBS and such foods are best kept to a minimum.

Dairy Products. Good sources of calcium and other necessary nutrients. "If they cause your symptoms to flare up, try decreasing the amount consumed at any one time. Yogurt can be a satisfactory substitute."

Fiber Foods. Dr. Cohen explains, "Dietary fiber, present in whole grain breads and cereals and in fruits and vegetables are helpful in lessening IBS symptoms. High-fiber diets keep the colon mildly distended, which helps prevent spasms. Some forms of fiber also keep water in the stools, thereby preventing formation of difficult stools. Doctors usually recommend that you eat just enough fiber so that soft, easily passed, painless movements are produced. High fiber diets may cause gas and bloating; however, over time these symptoms may dissipate as the digestive tract becomes adjusted to the increased fiber intake."

Eat Smaller Meals. Avoid cramping or diarrhea which may come from large meals. Smaller portions of foods at mealtimes, especially if the foods are low in fat and high in carbohydrates and protein may help to alleviate the symptoms."[80]

❧

CASE HISTORY—*Soothes "Angry Stomach" with Simple Lifestyle Changes*

Moving up the ladder of success gave Oliver E. more responsibilities, not to mention a bigger house (after the arrival of his third child), and heavier mortgage payments. As manager of a hotel chain, he was always on the go, had unrelieved tension, ate fast foods, with a minimum of nutrition but a maximum of fat! Often, he would gulp down huge amounts of food because he was in a hurry to go from one meeting to another. When he developed recurring cramps, irregular bowel habits and a feeling of "sour stomach" or bloating, he brought his problem to a gastroenterologist, who diagnosed his condition as irritable bowel syndrome. Immediately, he told Oliver E. to avoid any foods that caused symptoms. Less fat! That was an order! Smaller meals eaten in comfort . . . "or else don't eat at all!" Oliver E. was told to increase dietary fiber foods such as whole grains, bran cereals, brown rice, raw fruits (including skin and pulp), such as apples, grapes, peaches, pears, plums; some cooked fruit; more raw vegetables, such as broccoli, cabbage, carrots, celery, lettuce; some cooked high-fiber vegetables, such as Brussels sprouts, cauliflower, potatoes, squash, string beans, turnips.

He was told to handle stress better, to answer the call of nature promptly, to ease up on worrying and to avoid either very hot or very cold foods or beverages. Oliver E. followed the program . . . and in three weeks, his IBS symptoms subsided . . . vanished . . . and his painful intestinal contractions disappeared. These simple adjustments made him friends with his colon, and life became wonderful!

ITCHING

Symptoms

When you itch . . . you scratch. It feels sooooo good . . . and you pay the penalty when the irritation becomes worse. A vicious cycle! You scratch because you have a lump, bump or rash that has popped up somewhere on your body. You want relief . . . and quickly. The itch may be caused by an underlying condition, such as an allergy, shingles, chickenpox, hives, sunburn, diabetes, anemia, glandular malfunction. A medical practitioner can determine the underlying cause, which needs to be treated to help you find relief from itching.

Natural Remedies

You want help *right now*! Soothe your itch with these quick-acting, external natural remedies.

Ice Cools that Itch. Soak a towel in ice water and place it over the itching area. Repeat as often as desired. Or else, apply an ice pack. For overall itching, ease yourself into a tub of cold water and remain immersed until you feel better.

Oatmeal Soothes that Itch. Pour two cups of colloidal oatmeal (available at health stores or pharmacies) into a tub of tepid water, and remain immersed for about 20 minutes. (*Colloidal* means the oatmeal has been ground into a fine powder and remains suspended in water.)

Cotton Comforts that Itch. Whatever the cause of your itching, cotton clothing is more comforting than polyester or wool. Best to **AVOID** synthetics or itchy fabrics. Clothing that is too tight or poorly fitting can also cause itching. Cotton and comfort are two keys to relief from itching.

Cool Milk Takes Sting Out of Itch. Pour some cold milk into a glass with ice cubes. Let it remain for five minutes. Soak a thin piece of cotton in the mixture, and apply it to the itching area for three minutes. Resoak the cloth and continue reapplying for about 15 minutes. Helps take the "bite" out of the itch.

Beware of Quick or Sudden Temperature Changes. Going from the hot outdoors to the cold air-conditioned indoors, or even from a hot shower into a colder room, can cause an itching reaction as your skin and nerves try to adjust. **AVOID** these extremes. The same applies to water temperatures when you wash up. From hot to cold can be a shock to your skin and bring on a protesting itch. Easy does it as you move from comfortably warm to comfortably cool.

Ice Cube Treatment. For an agonizing itch that calls for instant relief, rub an ice cube over the area. The cold shrinks the blood vessels and keeps them from opening or swelling.

Five Ways to Resist Itching and Scratching. Nip the itch in the bud . . . before it starts. Five ways include: (1) **AVOID** rapid changes in temperature. (2) **AVOID** any violent exercise that provokes sweating. (3) **AVOID** rough, scratchy, tight clothing, especially woolens. (4) **AVOID** excessive use of soaps, hot water, and other cleansing procedures that could be abrasive and remove natural oils from your skin. (5) **AVOID** emotional upsets, which could provoke itching.

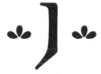

JET LAG

Symptoms

A temporary decline in physical and psychological well-being experienced by travelers who have rapidly crossed several time zones. Tiredness, irritation, stomach upset, headache are typical symptoms. Why does it happen? Your body clock—that internal timekeeper that governs your body's daily or circadian rhythms—is not synchronized with the time in the new environment. Traveling from coast to coast in the United States throws it off by three hours; flying to Europe puts you at least six hours out of synch; jetting to the Orient can throw you off by as many as 12 hours.

Circadian rhythms control your daily cycles of sleep, hunger, cardiovascular activity, body temperature, alertness, energy, and virtually every other bodily function, as these fluctuate through the 24-hour day. Eastward or westward jet travel has the effect of shortening or lengthening that day. And the more time zones you cross, the greater the discrepancy between the actual time and your internal time—that which is perceived by your master timekeeper called the hypothalamus (located in a brain structure). Therefore, to avoid or minimize jet lag, you need to adjust your biological clock.

Natural Remedies

To help reduce jet lag, here are some guidelines as offered by William C. Dement, M.D., Ph.D., Professor of Psychiatry and Behavioral Sciences and Director of the Sleep Disorders Center at Stanford University School of Medicine, in Palo Alto, California:

1. Try to **AVOID** a severe sleep deficit. Plan your flight to arrive in the new location before bedtime. Go to bed at the appropriate local time. When traveling to Europe, this means taking a morning rather than an overnight flight. On the other hand, you probably won't be sleepy at bedtime because it's six or more hours earlier than your usual time for sleep. Using the opposite strategy and missing a night's sleep for overnight travel may make you feel worse, but when it's bedtime in Europe, you'll

be ready to sleep—that is, if you've succeeded in staying awake all day.

2. Try to break up a very long flight, such as one to the Orient or Australia, with a one-day layover at an intermediate point. *Example*: If possible, make a rest stop for one day in Hawaii.

3. When business travel requires a brief stay in a distant time zone, try, if possible, to stick to home time. Schedule business meetings or work sessions during your home-time peak hours.

4. On excursions of more than a few days, it's best to adopt the new local time immediately upon your arrival. Schedule meals, work or touring, exercise, and sleep appropriately.

5. Spend time out of doors the first few days in order to expose yourself to sunlight in the new time zone, as this may help readjust your circadian rhythms.

6. If time permits, allow yourself two days to adjust to a new time zone, before starting an important work assignment or a rigorous touring schedule.

7. If possible, begin to preadapt to the new time zone for a few days before your departure. If you're going to be traveling eastward, try to eat your meals and go to bed one hour earlier each night for the three or four days immediately preceding your trip. Get up early in the mornings and into bright light or sunlight, but avoid sunlight in the afternoon or evenings before your departure because it will delay bodily rhythms, so that the need to sleep comes later.

8. Avoid overeating. Heavy foods place extra strain on your digestive system; your stomach is out of cycle anyway.

9. Drink lots of water and juices on the plane. It is unwise to drink alcohol because in combination with the pressurized air, it will cause dehydration.

10. To minimize fatigue, avoid cramped positions on the plane. Take regular walks in the aisles; exercise as space permits.[81]

Which Direction Influences Jet Lag? Most people have an easier time flying east to west (when they initially will experience a longer day), than west to east (when the first day is cut short), presumably because the natural circadian rhythm is really about 25, not 24 hours long; it is easier to adjust to the longer day than to the shorter one. *Remedy*: Based on his studies of the effects of daylight on a hormone called melatonin, which may be your body's main timekeeper, Dr. Alfred Lewy of the Oregon Health Sciences University, in Portland, suggests,

"When flying east to west, when you arrive, stay outside in the late afternoon. When flying west to east, when you arrive, go outside early in the morning for several hours."[82]

Visualization Eases Symptoms. Help your body speedily readjust to new time zones with a simple visualization *remedy*. Create mental images of what you would be doing at a given time, when you are already at your destination. Think pleasant, positive thoughts, or make plans for what you will be doing upon arrival and for several days afterwards.

Avoid Smoking. The accumulation of carbon monoxide in your blood combined with the effects of an altitude of 5,000 feet (the altitude to which the cabin is pressurized) is equivalent to the fatigue from lack of oxygen experienced at 10,000 feet. Keep away from others who smoke.

Eat Lightly. At 37,000 feet, the air in a plane is dry and thin, and your body works much harder at each function than at ground level. Watch how airplane personnel eat—moderately . . . and they work hard on the plane. Eat salads, fish, chicken or fruit. Avoid heavy meats, refined starches, and sweet desserts. If you take a night flight, eat before you fly, then avoid the meal served; put on eye shades and simulate a normal bedtime on the plane. It works!

And . . . enjoy the relaxation and solitude. It will help you adjust to the change in time zones all the easier.

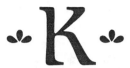

KIDNEYS

Symptoms

The kidneys are situated at the back of your abdomen, below your diaphragm, one on each side of your spine. Trouble starts when a grain of some hard substance—perhaps only a mineral—gets caught in the kidney. Urine crystallizes around it. The stone grows, and the pain tells you it is there. The pain of a kidney stone begins in your back. As the stone works its way through your urinary tract, the pain follows right along. Various over-the-counter medications, such as ibuprofen or aspirin, are available to reduce the pain, but when the drugs wear off, the pain is felt again. A stone may occasionally be passed off via urine. Or else, it may be removed by using electricity, ultrasound, or having it shattered by electrically-generated or laser-generated shock waves, while you sit anesthetized in a tub of water. These methods will pulverize as many as 99 percent of all stones. To cope with this disorder, you want to take better care of your kidneys, the filtering system of your body.

Natural Remedies

A set of healing remedies are suggested by Dr. Brian L.G. Morgan of the Institute of Human Nutrition at the Columbia University College of Physicians and Surgeons, in New York City:

Drink Lots of Liquids. Fluids help dilute your urine and prevent substances such as calcium oxalate from becoming concentrated enough to form crystals in the urine. At least four quarts of liquids daily will help keep your kidneys healthy.

Limit Vitamin C. If you have calcium oxalate kidney stones, restrict intake of vitamin C. This vitamin participates in the production of oxalate; it converts glyoxalate to oxalate which could form into stones. A general safety limit would be 3,000 to 4,000 milligrams daily, but over that amount could increase oxalate production and the risk of calcium oxalate stones. It is not likely you can overload on vitamin C from foods, so you should limit your use from any supplements.

Restrict Oxalate-High Foods. Dr. Morgan notes that "approximately 10 percent of the oxalate in the urine is derived from the diet." Ordinarily, it is given off in the wastes. "But if you have a fat malabsorption disorder, the fat you eat will combine with the calcium in foods, and both will be excreted in the stool. As a result, dietary oxalate will be left calcium-free and will be absorbed into your system. Since the oxalate cannot be broken down in the body, it is dispatched to the kidneys to be excreted in the urine, where it can combine with calcium to form calcium oxalate stones." Typical oxalate-rich foods to restrict include: beans, mustard greens, okra, beets, celery, chocolate, cocoa, spinach, tea, to name a few.

Vitamin B_6. This vitamin reduces the body's production of oxalate by as much as 50 percent. Dr. Morgan suggests, "Take a 100 to 200 milligram daily supplement of vitamin B_6 to reduce the amount of oxalate excreted into the urine and thereby reduce the risk of calcium oxalate stones."

Vitamin A. A deficiency could change the lining of the urinary tract and lead to calcium deposition and production of kidney stones. Dr. Morgan recommends 5,000 international units of vitamin A daily.

Keep Protein to a Minimum. There appears to be a link between kidney stone formation and the quantity of protein consumed. Protein increases the presence of acid, calcium, and phosphorus in the urine. This may predispose to stone formation. Dr. Morgan suggests no more than six ounces of protein-rich foods per day.

What About Calcium? The least important factor in the development of kidney stones is calcium. If your urine has unusually high levels of calcium, Dr. Morgan advises limiting calcium intake to 800 milligrams per day. Since you may risk developing osteoporosis, discuss your calcium needs with your health practitioner. "Oxalate excretion is a bigger factor in calcium oxalate stone production."

Cut Down on Salt. Salt is excreted along with calcium, which could cause a deficiency. Salt also irritates the kidneys. Reduce salt intake to two or three grams a day—about two teaspoons.[83]

Cranberry Juice May Be Helpful. A natural *remedy* calls for cranberry juice to help protect against kidney problems. Folklore has it that cranberries are acidic, so the juice will acidify the urine and discourage calcium stones from forming. You would need to drink a large quantity of cranberry juice to create any beneficial reaction. Still, you need a lot of fluid so you could include this juice as part of your natural remedy program for kidney health.

Fish Oils for Kidney Health. Patrick Quillin, Ph.D., R.D. Professor at UCLA tells us, "Eicosapentaenoic acid (EPA) from fish oil may improve the overall health of the kidneys. A variety of valuable prostaglandins, which help to regulate the kidneys, are readily produced from EPA. During pregnancy, a woman's body adds about 50 percent more to her existing fluid volume. Under this stress, sometimes the kidneys begin mistakenly to dump large amounts of protein into the urine. This condition, proteinuria, can sometimes be prevented or treated with EPA. EPA holds great potential in treating a wide variety of kidney diseases."[84]

Eicosapentaenoic acid or EPA is a fat that is valuable for keeping blood vessels healthy and the immune system functioning. It is available as a supplement; it is also found in seafood.

KNEE HURTS

Symptoms

You have 187 joints in your body—but the knee seems to become injured more than any of the others. You abuse your knees more than you think, especially when you climb stairs, scrub floors, participate in sports, bump against hard objects, not to mention poor posture. A common ailment is "runner's knee," a catchall term for all knee problems associated with running . . . but they can strike non-runners. For example, "housemaid's knee" can afflict any man or woman who spends much time on the knees, such as in laying floors, leaning against the rungs of a ladder while painting, working in a garden. The *problem* involves inflammation of the bursa in front of the kneecap. The tendons of the knees may also be hurt. In severe attacks, it may be painfully difficult to bend the knee.

Natural Remedies

For most knee hurts, ice is a soothing natural remedy. Lowell Scott Weil, D.P.M., Director of the Sports Medicine Center for the Scholl College of Podiatric Medicine in Chicago, Illinois and team podiatrist for the Chicago Bears, suggests,

"Ice cubes are ideal for applying to any sore area. Have some water-filled Dixie cups in the freezer for emergencies. For sore knees and muscles, keep some water-soaked Ace bandages in the freezer." She also suggests, "Following ice therapy, stretch a stiff or sore muscle to bring back range of motion." The stretching should be gradual and not jerky. Tight muscles will respond more quickly to a gentle stretching.[85]

Ice and Heat Remedy. Icing an inflamed knee joint for 20 minutes at a time, three or four times a day is often recommended for the first 48 hours. Thereafter apply heat—moist heat is best, and even a hot shower can help—for 15-minute intervals three times a day.

Common and Uncommon Knee Hurts and Remedies

Housemaid's Knee (Prepatellar Bursitis). Pain at front of knee; swelling, limited movement. *Remedy*: Rub ice on the knee until numb. Use protective pads on the knee if kneeling.

Runner's Knee (Chondromalacia Patellae). Kneecap pain when bending. Locking or grinding sensation; occasional swelling, quick fatigue, and weakness. *Remedy*: Avoid activities that call for bending of knee; use cold packs to ease pain.

Jumper's Knee (Patellar Tendinitis). Pain in front of the knee; swelling, redness, and warmth. *Remedy*: Rub with ice until numb. Use elastic knee supports. Avoid jumping!

Sprain (Torn Ligaments). Localized or diffuse pain. Instability, swelling, loss of motion. *Remedy*: Immobilize your knee with brace or crutches. Use cold packs or ice.

Iliotibial-Band Friction Syndrome. Burning pain on borders of the knee at the end of the thighbone after vigorous walking or activity. Some swelling. *Remedy*: Rub with ice until numb. Use corrective footwear.

To help protect against knee hurts, here are suggestions offered by James M. Fox, M.D., an orthopedic surgeon, Director of the Center for the Disorders of the Knee in Van Nuys, California:

1. Lose overweight, especially if you participate in vigorous activities. It will take much pressure off your knees.
2. Minimize squatting or excessive stair climbing because it puts a force four to seven times your weight across your kneecap. The stress between kneecap and thigh can be more than 2,000 pounds when you stand up. If you have to work below your waist, sit on the floor or use a stool.

3. Gardening? Put a foam cushion beneath your knees and keep shifting your weight. Keep changing your leg positions.

4. Do not walk in thinly soled shoes or high heels. "The most encouraging boon to knee joints in walking cities has been the number of women who wear walking shoes to work and brown-bag their high heels," says Dr. Fox. "Walking shoes should be well-cushioned, especially at the heel, and not overly stretched."

5. If you must sit for a period of time, change your position. "Cross and uncross your legs, slide forward in your seat, stretch your legs. Whenever possible, get up and walk around every 35 or 40 minutes."

6. If you do fast walking, be aware that hyperextending your legs—straining them to an abnormal degree—will stretch the tendons in the back of your knee and give you an ache. **TIP:** For normal walking or running, keep your knees slightly bent.

7. If your knee suddenly starts to hurt while you are in an activity, stop right away. "Do not try to work through the pain. You are likely to compound the damage. Instead, follow a simple first-aid *remedy* known by the acronym RICE: Rest, get off your feet. Ice the knee. Compression, or wrapping the knee gently. Elevate the leg," advises Dr. Fox.[86]

CAUTION: Seek medical help without delay if you feel numbness or tingling in your feet or toes; or if your knee is painful or swollen and especially if you feel something moving abnormally inside your knee. If you heard a "pop" inside your knee when the injury happened, medical help should be prompt to avoid serious damage.

❧ L ❧

LACTOSE INTOLERANCE

Symptoms

The inability to digest significant amounts of lactose is called lactose intolerance. In order to digest milk and dairy products, which are rich in *lactose*, your body needs an intestinal enzyme called *lactase*. If you have reduced levels of this enzyme, the undigested milk sugar sits in your large intestine and causes distressing symptoms. These include nausea, cramps, bloating, gas, and diarrhea. The symptoms begin about 30 minutes to two hours after eating or drinking foods that contain lactose. The severity of symptoms varies, depending on the amount of lactose that each individual can tolerate.

Some causes of lactose intolerance are well-known. For instance, certain digestive diseases and injuries to the small intestine can reduce the amount of enzymes produced. There may be inflammatory bowel disease, ulcerative colitis, malabsorption syndrome, or a recent intestinal infection. Certain ethnic groups are more widely affected than others.

Should you eliminate dairy products? Doing so could cause a serious calcium deficiency. You need this mineral for heartbeat regulation, blood clotting, nerve transmission, regulation of blood pressure—and also to protect against osteoporosis, a serious bone-thinning and potentially crippling *problem* that afflicts at least one out of every four women over age 50. You can manage milk with some adjustments, even with a deficiency of lactase.

Natural Remedies

Gary M. Gray, M.D., Professor of Medicine and Director of the Division of Gastroenterology at Stanford University Medical School, in California has these suggestions:

1. When trying to find your level of tolerance, it is best to begin with small amounts of lactose-containing foods. Aged cheeses (cheddar and Swiss) are very low in lactose. If these are well tolerated, moderate amounts of a cultured milk product (yogurt) may be added.

2. Divide the amount of milk, or other dairy products normally consumed, into small servings and eat them throughout the day. For example, two cups of milk per day can be consumed by dividing them into six servings of one-third cup each. A portion can be taken with each meal and the remainder with snacks. In this way, you can still obtain the valuable nutrients without the unpleasant symptoms.

3. Cultured buttermilk often appears to cause fewer symptoms than other types of milk. Sweet acidophilus milk, however, contains the same amount of lactose as other liquid milks and must be consumed in small quantities, as described above.

4. Milk-containing foods consumed hot are often better tolerated than cold ones.

5. An enzyme product, which is available in many health food stores, and pharmacies, converts the lactose to lactase and makes digesting milk more comfortable with few or no symptoms. When several drops of the enzyme preparation are mixed with a quart of milk and then refrigerated for 24 hours, about 70 percent of the lactose in the milk will have been predigested. The process can be speeded up if the milk is heated to 90°F. before the enzyme is added. The enzyme-treated milk can then be used in any way that ordinary milk is used. It will not be changed by heating. However, lactose-digested milk tastes sweeter than ordinary milk because the component sugars, glucose and galactose, taste sweeter than lactose. (Diabetics should consult their physicians before using lactase-treated milk.)[87]

Watch for Hidden Lactose. Many foods may contain lactose even in small amounts. These include: bread and other baked goods; processed breakfast cereals; instant potatoes, soups, and breakfast drinks; margarine; lunch meats (other than kosher); salad dressings; candies and other snacks; mixes for pancakes, biscuits, cookies, etc.; so-called non-dairy products such as powdered coffee creamer and whipped toppings may also include milk-derived lactose. **TIP:** Lactose is used as the base for many prescription drugs and over-the-counter medicines, especially in products for stomach acid and gas! Ask your pharmacist about the amounts of lactose in the product.

Read Labels. Look for more than milk or lactose among the contents. Be alert to such words as whey, curds, caseinate, lactoglobulin, and milk byproducts. Any of these words on a label indicates the item contains lactose.

Alternative Calcium Sources. These include soy milk, salmon with bones, sardines, tofu, bok choy, collards. But these may not give you the RDA of 1,000 milligrams. You may want to take a supplement!

Drink Milk with Solid Foods. Never drink milk alone! Take with solid food; this reduces the rate at which the milk passes down the digestive tract for intestinal absorption. Therefore, whatever lactase is present is better able to digest the milk. **TIP:** Milk taken with a whole grain cereal and fresh fruit at breakfast should improve lactose absorption by at least 60 percent. So . . . you can have your milk and drink it, too!

LIVER

Symptoms

Located behind the lower ribs on the right side of your abdomen, your liver is the largest organ in your body, weighing about three pounds and is roughly the size of a football. It plays a key role in converting food into essential substances of life. Your liver processes nutrients absorbed from the digestive tract into forms that are easier for the rest of your body to use. In essence, your liver can be considered your body's refinery. When something goes wrong with the liver, symptoms and signs of illness include: jaundice, or abnormally yellow discoloration of the skin and eyes; it is often the only sign of liver trouble. Look for dark urine, nausea, vomiting and/or loss of appetite, abdominal swelling, prolonged generalized itching, unusual change of weight, abdominal pain, sleep disturbances, mental confusion and coma, fatigue or loss of stamina, and loss of sexual drive or performance. *Liver Diseases*: viral hepatitis, cirrhosis, gallstones, alcohol-related disorders, cancer.

Natural Remedies

To keep your liver in good condition, nutrition forms a good foundation for providing certain elements.

Vitamins —optimal intake of vitamin A will help protect against the formation of tough, fibrous tissue symptomatic of cirrhosis. Vitamin E is also essential in helping to nourish cells of the liver.

Minerals —zinc helps build resistance to many liver disorders. Iron and copper will help nourish the cells of the liver.

TIPS: Fresh foods are a good source of nutrients; supplements should be optimal but not excessive to protect against stress on the liver. Avoid tobacco, alcohol, environmental irritants. Restrict salt to decrease fluid retention (edema). Plan a meal program around foods that are low in fat and high in fiber.

Iron? Easy Does It! Excessive iron supplementation may cause problems. An overload stored in the liver may lead to *hemosiderosis* (iron overload) and *hemochromatosis* (approaching point of damage). Symptoms of such disorders include bronzing of the skin, diabetes, enlarged heart, cardiac arrhythmias, abdominal pain. Each person reacts differently, but iron should be obtained from foods, for the most part.

Vegetables that Offer Healing Iron. These include carrots, potatoes, beets, pumpkin, broccoli, cauliflower, cabbage, turnips, tomatoes. *Important Benefit*: These foods are rich in ascorbic acid, citric acid, and malic acid, which boost iron absorption—a double-bonus for your liver.

"Poor" Iron Foods: Certain vegetables are nourishing with other nutrients but do not promote iron absorption because they contain phytate, a compound that blocks iron transmission; they are lentils, beet greens, butter beans and (sorry, Popeye!) spinach!

LOW BACK PAIN

Symptoms

Shooting spasms, muscular stiffness, cramped tightness are all symptoms of low back or lumbar pain. Waitresses on their feet all day, executives confined to long hours hunched over a desk, workers who lift and carry supplies—all are special targets for low back pain. Carrying heavy briefcases and wearing high heels can increase the likelihood. Your lumbrosacral joints are easily strained when excessive stresses of any kind are placed on the spine. Poor posture, incorrect sleeping or sitting positions, excessive fatigue are among the more common causes of low back pain.

An upright position puts constant pressure on the spongy, round, shock-absorbing disks between the stacked portions of the backbone, particularly those in the lower back. Poor body carriage, disuse of the muscles that help support the spine can also contribute to low back problems.

Natural Remedies

Most low back pain comes from poor posture and incorrect body mechanics (as in lifting and carrying). Dr. Jack Soltanoff, Doctor of Chiropractic, in West Hurley, New York, suggests these few simple rules to follow to ease occurrence of low back pain:

Standing and Walking. Flatten out the arch (lordosis) in the small of your back (lumbar spine). Bend your knees slightly, tuck in your buttocks or "tail;" and tuck in your stomach (abdominal) wall—and don't suck in or tighten your abdominal wall. Don't hold your breath while you do this.

- Stand with your back against a wall, at first, and try to make the small of your back touch the wall when you tuck in your tail and belly. Keep this posture when you walk away from the wall.

- If you have a large stomach up front, or if you're pregnant, you may have to bend your knees more than slightly to get the proper tucking in of your tail and your abdominal wall.

- Practice walking with your tail and belly tucked in. You'll feel stiff and awkward at first but in a short time you'll do it with ease.

- Avoid bending forward over any work you do while standing, whether at a sales counter or at the ironing board—or when using a paint brush or the vacuum cleaner. If necessary, bend your knees, not your back, to get down closer to your work.

Lifting and Carrying. Bend your knees instead of your back when you pick anything up or put it down, no matter how heavy or light the object is. When you carry a heavy object, use two hands and keep it close to your waist.

- When lifting or carrying, give special emphasis to keeping your tail and belly tucked in, and use your legs to take the load.

- When lifting any object, heavy or light, get close to it before you bend your knees to pick it up. And keep in mind that raising a window sash is the same as lifting an object.

- When carrying a heavy object, exaggerate the bend in your knees and the tucking in of your tail. Don't reach out to put the object down. Walk up close and bend your knees to put it down.

- Avoid putting heavy objects on any surface higher than your waist.

If you must push or pull a heavy object, bend your knees, tuck in your tail and *push* rather than pull. Also, bending over to dry your feet, or to step into your trousers or pantyhose, can be just as risky as bending over to pick up a 50-pound bag of fertilizer.

- Tucking in your tail for all of these activities will become easier if you practice tightening your buttocks muscles and keep them tightened while tucking in. You know how to "make a muscle" in your arm; do the same to make the muscles hard in your seat.

Give Yourself a Back Rub. Dr. Jack Soltanoff suggests you apply a lotion to your hands and then stroke gently along the tops of your shoulders and up and down your back. "You may feel areas that are tight. These areas need more attention. By rubbing around and pressing into those tight spots, you can relieve tension and stiffness in your lower back."

Quick Helps for Low Back Pain. Dr. Soltanoff suggests, "Lie down on your side and pull your knees upward toward your chest. Rest for about 15 minutes. Or else, bow your head backward to reverse the forward curve. Focus on standing tall in order to keep your spine from sagging. Tuck your hips under a little in order to flatten out your lower back."

Be Sure to Rest. When you feel a pain, be sure to rest. Take the pain off your lower back with comforting relaxation.

Moist Heat Detoxifies Congestion. "Wrap a hot water bottle (filled with hot faucet water) in a piece of woolen blanket that has been wrung out in hot water. Both your back and the bottle should then be covered with a sheet of plastic in order to hold in the heat. Let the application remain on the aching part until the heat cools off. Reapply it about four times a day," says Dr. Soltanoff. CAREFUL: Do not use boiling hot water since it may penetrate the towels and cause a burn. Water heated to about 125°F will be hot enough. *Benefit:* This moist heat application stimulates blood circulation; it aids in the removal of waste products and accumulating tissue fluids.

And be careful to avoid chilling a muscle by direct exposure to the cooling drafts of a fan or an air-conditioner, especially when you are perspiring.

"The key to easing most lower back pain is a well-developed trunk and torso—one that maintains balanced strength between the muscles of the front of the trunk (abdominals) and the back of the trunk (erector spinae muscles). Abdominal strength helps you control excessive lordosis, or arching of the lower back, which is one of the main causes of back pain," says Dr. Soltanoff.[88]

Sleeping Tips. The proper way to sleep is either on your back with your head and knees propped up or on your side with your head propped up slightly. Do **not** sleep on your stomach as this will cause your spine to sway in the middle.

LUNG DISORDERS

Symptoms

Difficulties in breathing, constant allergic reactions, choking, sputtering, swallowing problems. Many lung disorders are traced to air pollution which comes in many disguises:

Ozone —the most widespread pollutant. Unlike the natural ozone gas in the upper atmosphere, which shields the earth from damaging ultraviolet rays, the ozone gas at ground level is a health hazard. Ozone forms when nitrogen oxides and volatile organic compounds, two other gaseous pollutants, react under the influence of sunlight. Nitrogen oxides are released by motor vehicles and industrial plants; volatile organics come from such diverse sources as backyard barbecues and dry cleaners.

Smog —a complex brew of pollutants including carbon monoxide, nitrogen oxides, sulfur oxides, particulates and ozone. These pollutants come from motor vehicles, industrial plants, electric utilities; organic vapors given off by paints, dry-cleaning chemicals, starter fluid used to ignite charcoal, and even the fermentation process used in bakeries contribute to smog formation.

CAUTION: At highest risk are people with chronic respiratory illness, anemia or cardiovascular problems. Allergy attacks will worsen and occur more frequently when such persons are exposed to pollution. Damage to bronchial passages can lead to lung lesions and lung disease.

Natural Remedies

You need to boost your immune system to protect against tissue breakdown because of the corrosive damage of chemical pollutants in the air you breathe.

Vitamins Improve Lung Function. Vitamin B_6 (pyridoxine) and vitamin C appear to strengthen the cells and tissues of the respiratory system housing the lungs. These nutrients help ease bronchial spasms while reducing sensitivity to offensive, inhaled invaders. They are available as supplements. A rule of thumb would be 100 milligrams of vitamin B_6 daily and 2,000 milligrams of vitamin C daily.

Avoid Smoking. You don't need more chemicals entering your system. Tobacco smoke dissolves your neutrophils, the disease-fighting warriors of your white blood cells, and renders your lungs susceptible to injury. Keep away from others who smoke, since this "passive smoke" can cause as much harm as if you smoked!

Keep Airways Free of Toxins. In an area you know has fresh air (country, or near the ocean, or a large body of water), practice this simple lung-washing *remedy*: fill your lungs with air as you breathe in through your nose. Then blow out slowly through pursed lips. Do this for 30 minutes. You'll help keep your airways cleansed of toxins. Repeat several times a day.

Balance Breathing with Your Work. When you lift, exhale through pursed lips. When you have to climb stairs, exhale through pursed lips. And . . . inhale while you rest! This rhythm helps improve your lung function.

Wear Comfortable Clothes. To ease pressure on your lungs, wear comfortable clothing that permits your chest and abdomen to expand freely. No tight girdles, belts or bras. Women may want to wear more comfortable camisoles instead of bras. Men and women might opt for suspenders instead of tight belts.

Avoid Temperature Extremes. Blasts of cold air, excessive humidity, abrupt changes in seasons, all will upset your breathing. Keep away from such situations wherever possible.

Control Your Emotions. Fear, anger, frustration, coughing, shouting, temperamental behavior, and crying will also upset your respiration and cause lung distress. Be alert to stress-filled circumstances and sidestep them. You'll breathe a lot better!

LYME DISEASE

Symptoms

If a tick bites you, you may have to worry about more than just a bite. Some ticks carry Lyme disease, so named because it was first recognized in Old Lyme, Connecticut. It is a bacterial infection transmitted by tiny ticks that are usually carried by deer and mice. Usually the first sign of Lyme disease is a red circular rash around the tick bite. It is often accompanied by fever, fatigue, aches, and other flu-like miseries. In more advanced stages, it can cause arthritis, degeneration of cartilage, neurological problems. "Summer is the worst time for Lyme disease," notes Sidney Hurwitz, M.D., Clinical Professor of Pediatrics and Dermatology at Yale University School of Medicine, in New Haven, "During the summer months, people spend more time in the woods and tall grass where they can be exposed to the tick, and the number of cases of Lyme disease skyrockets. Although the disease can strike people of any age, 70 percent of its victims are children under 19, the age group most likely to be wandering through fields, tall grass or the woods. Not all ticks carry Lyme disease, so you shouldn't panic if you're bitten by a tick." But you should seek help!

Natural Remedies

Dr. Hurwitz offers these suggestions for those who spend time in the woods:

- When going into woods that could be tick-infested, wear a hat, a long-sleeved shirt and long pants that are tucked into stockings or boots.
- Wear shoes with closed toes.
- Know where ticks live: marshy places, woods and forests, bushes, shrubs, and long grass (even in your own backyard); stay off trails, avoid brushing against vegetation.
- Collared shirts help reduce the chance of a tick getting up onto your skin, since ticks generally crawl upwards.
- Wear-light-colored clothing to make ticks easier to find. Wear tightly-woven fabrics to make it more difficult for them to hold on to your clothing.
- Be careful: Ticks can be found nearly anyplace outdoors. People and pets can bring them indoors. Ticks wait on low vegetation for a host (human or animal) to pass by. Ticks do not have wings and cannot jump or fly; instead, they cling to humans or animals and crawl upwards to find a place to attach and feed.

How To Remove Ticks. Follow these instructions:

1. Use small, pointed tweezers.

2. Grasp as close as possible to the mouthparts—don't grasp the tick's body.

3. Pull the tick away from your skin—do not twist or jerk.

4. Pull gently but firmly until the tick releases its hold.

5. Save the tick in a small jar of alcohol for your physician's examination.

6. Wash your hands and the bite with soap and water.

Dr. Hurwitz tells us, "It is important to remove the *whole* tick. If mouthparts remain in your skin, disinfect the area with alcohol and consult your physician."

Check Symptoms: The first sign is usually a rash at the site of a tick bite, often accompanied by headache, low fever, fatigue and other flu-like symptoms. The rash expands over the course of days or weeks before it disappears. "If you experience clinging symptoms, you should seek prompt medical help. This is especially important if you have been diagnosed as having arthritis, neurological disorders and heart problems. Pregnant women are at special risk because of reports of miscarriages and the passing on of Lyme disease to the fetus."[89]

If you notice any secondary problems, such as stiffening and pain in one or more joints—most often the knee or ankle—see your physician without delay!

Lyme disease is serious, but it can be beaten!

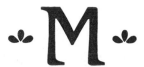

MEMORY

Symptoms

"What's your name again!" Or else, "Was that appointment for Tuesday or Thursday!" Then again, "I'm so sorry to be late for lunch. I completely forgot we had an appointment this afternoon." Memory lapses? Forgetfulness! In today's activity-filled lifestyle, it is not unusual to forget a few basics such as the name of someone you met a short while ago, or a few figures given to you an hour ago. But if you forget an important business or social appointment, you could be headed for embarrassment and trouble, too.

Natural Remedies

The following set of tricks stimulate an enzyme to manufacture acetylcholine, an important neurotransmitter that carries messages between neurons or brain cells. Neurotransmitters are abundant in your hippocampus, a small cluster of brain cells important in memory. Your goal is to jog your production of neurotransmitter chemicals so you can think more clearly and remember much better.

With the use of associate aids, such as making a rhyme for a person's name, an imprint is made in your brain. It stirs up neurotransmitter activation to give your hippocampus more memory recall. (Remember? You just read that!)

Here is a set of such natural remedies offered by Erwin DiCyan, Ph.D., Psychotherapist in Brooklyn, New York, who has helped many patients develop better memory power ranging from faces to entire pages and books. "Remember, you never lose the memory of something you learn. The problem lies in retrieving it." Here's how:

1. *Understand and Repeat.* Make sure you thoroughly understand the topic or event you need to remember. Then repeat or review, saying out loud to yourself, what you have just learned. ***Example:*** When introduced to someone, tack on the name to the "how do you do?" greeting. As often as possible, repeat the name during the conversation. You can better remember the name for future meetings.

2. *The Association Trick.* To remember something you have just learned, associate it with another item. Purchasing apples, bananas and eggplant becomes "Abe." Remembering Evelyn Zimmer becomes "EZ" or "easy." "Linkage helps recall names, dates, events, purchases."

3. *Use Familiar Rhymes.* Remember "Thirty days hath September"? It helped you remember how many days in the 12 months of the year. Use the same memory trick in current situations. *Example*: Do you move the clock ahead in the spring for daylight-saving time? The rhyme, "Spring forward, fall backward," jogs your memory. Make a simple rhyme and keep repeating until it can always be called into action.

4. *Make a Word out of Numbers.* Most telephone numbers or street addresses can be made into a word that's much easier to remember than figures. Example: 487-2263 spells "husband." Make two words if need be. Keep repeating it to help you remember the word-created number set.

5. *Correct Your Posture—Boost Your Memory.* Can't think straight? Your posture may be putting a crimp on the blood supply to your brain. Reason? Your brain requires up to 30 times more blood than other organs. But allowing your upper body to sag can create kinks in the spine that squeeze the two arteries passing through your spinal column to your brain, causing an inadequate blood supply. What happens? Fuzzy thinking and forgetfulness. So maintain good posture and improve your memory![90]

The Food that Improves Memory. Lecithin, often made from soy beans or sunflower seeds, is a prime source of phosphatidyl choline, a nutrient that helps nourish your brain enzymes, thereby stimulating them to release the all-*important* neurotransmitter that carries messages between your neurons. You may want to use several tablespoons of lecithin granules daily, in your whole grain breakfast cereal, to get your memory churning for the day (and night) ahead. Lecithin is available in many health stores.

Keep Your Mind Fit—Exercise It. Do this by memorizing something every day. Learn a new language. Play thinking games such as checkers, bridge, chess. Work on complicated crossword puzzles and word games. Give your mind a daily workout, and you'll have a healthy memory. Remember that!

MENOPAUSE

Symptoms

More popularly referred to as the "change of life," menopause comes from two Greek words meaning "to cease" and "month." Strictly speaking, menopause refers to the cessation of menstruation. It has a specific point in time: the last monthly period. For most women, menopause occurs at approximately age 51, but it may arrive earlier or later. Basically, the ovaries halt their production of the female hormone, estrogen. The most common symptom is the hot flash, a vasomotor disturbance triggered by altered levels of hormones. In most cases, the flash is accompanied by profuse perspiration. Women may experience an "aura" or uneasy feeling. The flash is often followed by chills and sometimes intense shivering, along with a feeling of constriction of the skin, which may last for a few hours. Flashes usually last for three to six minutes, but may also last up to one hour. With estrogen loss, there are vaginal changes such as shrinking, less elasticity, more susceptibility to infection. Bone mass thins, leading to osteoporosis. Overall, skin becomes drier as fertility ends. Emotional upset is common.

Natural Remedies

To cope with the "change," the basics call for

1. dressing in "layered" fashion to adjust to temperature changes;
2. AVOID hot environments—stay cool;
3. AVOID alcohol and caffeine, or keep them to a bare minimum;
4. drink adequate amounts of water, especially after exercise or strenuous work;
5. begin or continue a regular exercise program;
6. use relaxation techniques;
7. follow a low-salt program to avoid edema or water accumulating in the tissues;
8. you may need calcium supplements to help protect against osteoporosis;
9. keep yourself active via a hobby, gardening, crafts, lots of walking, dancing, nature hikes, as a means of avoiding depression and anger;

10. become selective about accomplishing tasks. Do one thing at a time to **AVOID** becoming too anxious.

Nutritional Boosters. Niels Lauersen, M.D., Professor of Obstetrics and Gynecology at Mt. Sinai Hospital, in New York City, tells of one patient, Ms. N. who was troubled with menopausal symptoms, especially stress. He felt she could be helped to reduce stress with vitamins and recommended she take one of the following each day: vitamin E, 800 to 1,000 units; vitamin D, 400 units; Calcium, 2,000 to 3,000 milligrams; vitamin B complex with vitamin B_6, 100 to 500 milligrams; Zinc, 50 milligrams; vitamin C, 1,000 milligrams.[91]

Vitamin E Soothes Symptoms. In various reports, vitamin E in amounts of 100 to 200 units daily may help relieve symptoms such as hot flashes. This vitamin controls production of prostaglandins, which cause certain types of discomfort.

Keep Yourself Active. At least 60 minutes of exercise daily will help ease symptoms. Exercise not only improves your emotional health, but also provides an overall feeling of contentment. Exercise increases brain concentrations of two *important* neurotransmitters: norepinephrine and serotonin, both needed to help you feel mentally and physically fit. **TIPS:** Try a 60-minute brisk walk every day. Also include aerobics, stretching exercises, especially yoga, which improves diaphragmatic breathing, so that you have less stress and can breeze through symptoms much more easily.

Keep Cool. Not only temperature, but emotionally. What causes upset and overheating? Stress? A hot meal? Spicy foods? Arguments? Work overload? Certain people or situations? Make every effort to avoid such "hot spots."

Smaller Meals Throughout the Day. Lighter eating means lighter symptoms. Spread meals out into six smaller offerings throughout the day, to help balance body temperature. And . . . lots and lots of cool water and juice is needed to control your temperature.

Hints, Tips, Suggestions. Be careful about drugs, such as antihistamines and decongestants, which dry out mucous membranes. Keep your weight down, to minimize symptoms exacerbated by obesity. Eat less food high in saturated and unsaturated fats. Avoid salt-cured, salt-pickled and smoked foods, such as sausages, smoked fish and ham, bacon, bologna and hot dogs. Eat less red meat. Avoid carbonated soft drinks, which contain phosphates that cause mineral imbalance associated with osteoporosis. Don't smoke, which causes not only cancer and heart disease, but brings on earlier menopause.

❦

CASE HISTORY—*Cools off Hot Flashes with Natural Remedies*

Knowing her "change" was approaching, Emma LaF. began to improve her basic health. She took the nutritional supplements recommended previously, became an exercise enthusiast, corrected her food program to boost fresh fruits, vegetables, whole grains, more poultry and seafood, and less red meats. Yes, Emma LaF. still had some symptoms but they were minimal because she prepared her body to meet the change . . . and it was a cool breeze!

MIGRAINE HEADACHES

Symptoms

Its name comes from the Greek word *hemikrania* or "half the head," which describes the locale of most migraines around the forehead, temple, ear, jaw, or eye. Migraine begins with lights, flashes, or with no warning, then evolves into dull, throbbing, recurring pain that is often incapacitating. There is head-splitting agony that lasts from two hours to a day. There is frequently accompanying anorexia, nausea, vomiting, mood changes, sensitivity to light and noise, cold hands and feet, upper respiratory congestion. There may be tingling or numbness in an arm or leg, restlessness and mental confusion. Attacks may be experienced three times a week . . . or three times a year. The frequency varies with each person.

Natural Remedies

Food allergy is one major cause. You may prevent and overcome migraine with some dietary adjustments.

Eliminate Tyramine Foods. A food substance that acts as a vasodilator, tyramine causes blood vessels to expand, boosts blood flow through blood vessels in the scalp to trigger a migraine. Tyramine is found in aged or ripened cheese, chicken and beef livers, eggplant, sour cream, salami, meat tenderizers, chocolate, red wines, caffeine-containing drinks, soy sauce. AVOID alcoholic beverages; dangerous ones are beer, sherry, Chianti, sauterne wines, and Reisling wine.

AVOID *Monosodium Glutamate.* You may be sensitive to MSG and develop "Chinese restaurant syndrome," which triggers migraine-like headache, chest tightness, burning sensation in the neck and forearms. TIP: Read packaged and processed foods labels to see if they contain MSG. When dining in Oriental restaurants, request that MSG be omitted, but you still have no assurance it will be done. (Many restaurants use processed ingredients that already have MSG added.)

Follow a Regular Schedule. Get up at the same time each morning. Eat meals at regular intervals. Go to sleep at the same time each night. You help regulate your blood sugar with this schedule, and this helps you avoid migraine and other discomforts.

Correct Sleeping Posture. Cramped, awkward positions, or even sleeping on your stomach can contract neck muscles and give you migraine. Train yourself to sleep on your back!

Hot or Cold Applications. Whatever makes you feel good! Apply cold (or comfortable heat) to your forehead or neck. If it works, do it often!

Keep Away from Cured Meats. They usually contain nitrates or preservatives that will dilate your blood vessels to give you a headache. Nitrates are usually found in luncheon and other cured meats, such as hot dogs, sausages, etc.

Herbal Pain-Killers. Quick relief is possible with these alternatives to chemicals or medications that may be upsetting.

Feverfew Leaf. Brew in a pot of water as you would tea. Add a bit of lemon juice and honey. Sip several cups a day.

Lavender-Valerian Tea. In combination, very soothing to ease stress accompanying migraine. Helps relax vascular contractions.

Chamomile Tea. Extremely soothing to ease pressures that trigger headaches. Helps take the "tightness" out of your head.

Correct Your Blood Sugar. Hypoglycemia can cause dilation of blood vessels in the head. It happens after a period without food: overnight, for example, or when a meal is skipped. If you wake up in the morning with a headache, you may be reacting to the low blood sugar caused by lack of food overnight. *Remedy*: Schedule smaller, more frequent meals. AVOID sugar. Balance complex carbohydrates with protein foods.

With these natural remedies, you will, in effect, "retrain" your blood vessels to react less strenuously to migraine-trigger factors.

MOTION SICKNESS

Symptoms

The French call it *mal de mer*, but even the most experienced sailors can have distress. In the air, it is airsickness. On land, it is car sickness. It all adds up to the same distress—a queasy, uneasy feeling. Your stomach churns and turns. You look and feel ill, on the verge of nausea, which impairs your sense of balance and equilibrium. Symptoms of motion sickness and dizziness appear when your central nervous system (brain and spinal cord) receives conflicting messages from your other systems (inner ears, eyes, skin, muscle-joint sensory receptors). Conflicting signals to your brain about the sensation of rotation may trigger a sense of spinning or vertigo, as well as nausea.

Natural Remedies

A set of remedies is suggested by the American Academy of Otolaryngology that helps most people:

1. Always ride where your eyes will see the same motion that your body and inner ears feel; for example, sit in the front seat of the car and look at the distant scenery; go up on the deck of the ship and watch the motion of the horizon; sit by the window of the airplane and look outside. TIP: In an airplane, choose a seat over the wings where the motion is the least.
2. Do not read while traveling if you are subject to motion sickness. Do not sit in a seat facing backwards.
3. Do not watch or talk to another traveler who is having motion sickness.
4. Avoid strong odors and spicy or greasy foods that do not agree with you (immediately before and during travel). Medical research has not yet investigated the effectiveness of such remedies as soda crackers or cola syrup over ice.

5. Avoid rapid changes in position, especially from lying down to standing up or turning around from one side to the other.

6. Avoid extremes of head motion (especially looking up) or rapid head motion (especially turning or twisting).

7. Eliminate or decrease use of products that impair circulation, such as nicotine, caffeine, and salt.

8. Minimize your exposure to circumstances that precipitate dizziness, such as stress and anxiety, or substances to which you are allergic.

Ginger Remedy. In a double-blind study at Brigham Young University, in Provo, Utah, Dr. Daniel B. Mowrey gave either Dramamine (a popular drug that prevents motion sickness) or a placebo, or ginger capsules to students susceptible to motion sickness. All were then blindfolded and rotated in a tilting chair for up to six minutes. Half the subjects given ginger lasted for the full six minutes. None of the subjects given Dramamine or the placebo could last the full six minutes of movement. Dr. Mowrey recommends two or three gelatin capsules, each containing about 500 milligrams of powdered ginger root, half an hour before the expected motion. *Note:* Ginger should be taken only in capsule form to **AVOID** burning the esophagus.[92] Ginger works by absorbing acids and blocking nausea in your gastrointestinal tract.

Refresh Your Nostrils. Unpleasant odors (engine fumes, decaying fish on ice, or even food ready to eat) can contribute to nausea. For relief, bring along large leaves of fresh angelica. Crush them during your journey, and breathe in the fragrance. The scent refreshes stale air and allays nausea. Wherever possible, you can deter symptoms with a breath of fresh air. On an airplane, turn on the overhead vent. Elsewhere, open a car window, or breathe in a sea breeze.

Look at Something Stationary. Balance your sensory network. The horizon that bobs, as on a boat, can be upsetting. Look at something stationary on the land or in the sky and stare at it!

Place Yourself Where There Is the Least Motion. In a car, sit in the front seat, looking ahead. Focus on distant objects rather than nearby ones moving past you. If not possible, close your eyes rather than peering at fast-moving scenery. **TIP:** In a bus, take the two seats just behind the front door. And . . . on a ship, remain amidships (preferably on deck). Try to get a cabin in the middle, at the waterline so you'll rock less.

MUSCLE INJURIES

Symptoms

A muscle spasm sends out waves of radiating hurt. Pain is a physical signal that something is wrong; your body has been subjected to some injury, some insult, and demands attention. If a muscle becomes overloaded with metabolic by-products, you feel pain. You lift a package that is too heavy, overdo it in physical activities, miscalculate and realize, too late, you don't know your own strength. Sprains and strains encompass a number of ailments including wrenched knees, tennis elbow, twisted ankles and sprained wrists. What is the difference between a sprain and a strain?

A *sprain* is caused by a twisting motion that rips or tears the ligaments that bind up the joints. A sprain generally takes longer to heal than a strain.

A *strain* or "pulled muscle" is any damage to a muscle or to the tendon that anchors the muscle. It is what you feel when you overexert your muscle. The muscle fibers become pulled, inflamed, or even torn. A strain usually afflicts an area near a joint but not in it. No matter what you call it, your muscle hurts and you want help . . . fast!

Natural Remedies

The basic four-step remedy for most injuries helps ease pain swiftly:

1. **ICE** should be applied to the injury immediately. This decreases the bleeding from injured vessels by causing them to constrict. The ice should be left on for 30 minutes, removed for 15 minutes and then reapplied. This may be repeated for up to three hours.

2. **COMPRESSION** limits the swelling, which can retard healing. This is accomplished by wrapping the strain or sprain snugly, but not too tightly, with an elastic bandage. **TIP:** The bandage may be applied over the ice.

3. **REST** is absolutely necessary to prevent continued exercise or movement that might extend the injury.

4. **HEAT** should be applied the next day or six to ten hours after the last ice treatment. This stimulates the blood flow, inhibits muscle cramps and relaxes tense muscles in the area of the injury.

TIP: Do not use the injured joint for a few days. Elevation (raising the injured arm or leg above the hard level) will help drain excess fluid from the affected area and speed healing.

Ice Is Natural Pain Reliever. For most muscle injuries, ice is the first line of defense against swelling. Wrap ice in a cloth or plastic bag and apply for 20 minutes at a time throughout the day. **CAREFUL:** Don't overdo it. More is not necessarily better. Ice will constrict your blood vessels, and it is unwise to keep them so tight for too long. You could hurt the viable tissue in that region. Instead, apply ice for 20 minutes . . . remove for 20 minutes . . . then apply again. You may do this throughout much of the day. **CAUTION:** If you have cardiovascular problems, diabetes or vascular disorders, you should use ice with much care and the approval of your health practitioner.

Healing Heat. For severe soreness or strain, you may want to alternate between ice and heat. Don't do it too soon or you may cause swelling of the injured area. Apply heat the easy way—in a warm bath, via a heating pad, a whirlpool. A 20 minute application helps dilate the cramped blood vessels and speed healing.

Rub Away Your Pain. Massage works to hasten the removal of metabolic by-products from the tissues by squeezing them out of the muscle fibers and back into the bloodstream for recirculation or elimination. Massage increases venous and lymphatic circulation, stimulates blood flow, and helps nourish muscle tissue, to increase joint mobility and flexibility. With one or both hands, rub the hurt. The muscle you are working on should always be relaxed. Work towards your heart in massage—always from the insertion of the muscle (the point farthest from the heart) to the origin (the point closest.) Stroke, knead and stroke. About 20 minutes will soothe the injury. Don't press too hard. Easy does it.

S-t-r-e-t-c-h. Simple stretching exercises . . . sitting or standing . . . that extend your limbs *comfortably* will help loosen the tightness and restore better flexibility and freedom from much pain. Do frequent stretching motions throughout the day.

Many muscle injuries develop when you push your body too far, too fast, too long. Know your limits and your body will resist the wrench of an agonizing muscle hurt!

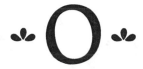

OBESITY

Symptoms

What is a healthy weight for you?

Healthy weight for adults means meeting these THREE conditions:

1) Your weight falls within the range for your height and age in the table. (*Note:* The lower weights in the ranges are best for most women, who have less muscle and bone than men.)

2) Your waist measure is smaller than your hip measure.

3) Your doctor has not advised you to gain or lose weight for some health reason.

If you don't meet these conditions, ask your doctor about how your weight may affect your health and what to do about it.

Natural Remedies

You will help reshape behavior by aiming for a balance between caloric intake and caloric expenditure. If you lead a moderatively active life, you need about 15 calories per pound to maintain your weight. *Example:* If you are 150 pounds, you need no more than 2,250 calories each day to maintain your weight. *Losing Weight:* To lose one pound, you need to burn 3,500 calories more than are consumed. **TIP:** Reduce calories by 500 per day and increase daily activity to burn off an additional 250 calories and you will lose about 1 ½ pounds per week. *Benefit:* Gradual weight loss promotes long-term loss of body fat, rather than just water weight that can be quickly regained.

Become More Physical. Regular aerobic exercise, such as brisk walking, jogging or swimming is a key factor in achieving permanent weight loss. Aerobic exercise works the body's large muscles, such as your heart, and should be moderately vigorous, but not exhausting, to

SUGGESTED WEIGHTS FOR ADULTS

Height without shoes	Weight in pounds	Without clothes
	19 to 34 years	35 years and over
5'0"	97–128	108–138
5'1"	101–132	111–143
5'2"	104–137	115–148
5'3"	107–141	119–152
5'4"	111–146	122–157
5'5"	114–150	126–162
5'6"	118–155	130–167
5'7"	121–160	134–172
5'8"	125–164	138–178
5'9"	129–169	142–183
5'10"	132–174	146–188
5'11"	136–179	151–194
6'0"	140–184	155–199
6'1"	144–189	159–205
6'2"	148–195	164–210
6'3"	152–200	168–216
6'4"	156–205	173–222
6'5"	160–211	177–228
6'6"	164–216	182–234

be most effective. **TIP:** Plan to exercise at least six times per week, for at least 30 minutes each time. **CAUTION:** Any amount less will not burn off calories—so no cheating!!

Exercise: Appetite Remedy. Exercise not only burns calories, it increases your body's metabolic rate and actually decreases your appetite. Exercise has an emotional benefit. It improves your sense of well-being and eases stress—which often leads to compulsive or nervous over-eating.

When exercise is used with a weight-losing program, a higher percentage of net weight loss is adipose (fat) tissue. This remedy provides optimal calorie and fat-burning benefits and minimal stress on bones and joints.

Adjust Your Behavior Pattern. Barbara DeBetz, M.D., Assistant Clinical Professor of Psychiatry at Columbia University, College of Physicians and Surgeons, in New York City, calls for a change in attitude

FITNESS IS FUN . . . AND SLIMMING

Expenditures in Calories by a 150 Pound Person

Activity	Total Calories Per Hour
Ballroom dancing	125–310
Walking slowly (2½ mph)	210–230
Brisk walking (4 mph)	250–345
Jogging (6 mph)	315–480
Cycling (9 mph)	315–480
Tennis	315–480
Basketball	480–625
Aerobic Dancing	480–625
Swimming	480–625
Cross-Country Skiing	480–625

when losing weight. "When you start a diet, you begin to fight food—you think 'don't eat this, don't eat that, *don't, don't, don't.*' And it's just basic human behavior that the more you say 'don't do something,' the more you'll want to do it." As a psychiatrist and bariatrician (weight loss specialist), Dr. DeBetz has helped countless patients lose weight—and just as importantly, keep it off." She offers these behavior modification programs to put you in control of your appetite:

Touch Control Signal. The technique involves looking upwards, closing your eyes, then gently touching some area of your face with the tip of your forefinger. As you do so, repeat these phrases, concentrating on the word "body." Say: "For my body, overeating is an insult. I need my body to live. I owe my body this respect and attention." Dr. DeBetz explains, "It's like a braking device. The touch-control signal helps you stop and consider what you are doing; it helps shift your focus from food to your body."

Enjoy Your Food. Dr. DeBetz advises, "While you eat, do not watch TV, do not read or do anything else. Otherwise, you won't be aware of what and how much you eat and will not know when you've had enough."

Is It Physical or Emotional Hunger? Here's a clue—physical hunger is a gnawing sensation, while emotional hunger is a craving for a specific food. Make up a list of alternative activities to turn to when you're emotionally hungry. "You might exercise, listen to music, go to the movies, call a friend, take a warm bath," suggests Dr. DeBetz.

Exercise Your Mind. Follow these three emotional exercises each day. "They are what I call my three STOPlines. I ask people to recite them five times daily or whenever the idea of food lures them to break their diet. They are: (1) For my body, overeating is an insult and a poison. (2) I need my body to live. (3) I owe my body this respect and protection."

Fat-Fighting Remedies

If you eat out of Frustration, Anxiety and Tension, you will end up being F A T. Dr. DeBetz helps you avoid this threat with a set of easy and effective fat-fighting and slimming natural remedies:

1. Always serve food on smaller individual plates. Serving "family style" encourages larger portions and second helpings.
2. Clear leftovers directly into the garbage or to your family pet. Saving them for tomorrow's lunch is, in reality, plotting for to-night's nibbling.
3. Know your "danger times" for nibbling. Plan in advance any activity that will divert you from the refrigerator during that time span.
4. Never watch TV, read or talk on the phone while eating. This will detract from your oral satisfaction and leave you feeling "cheated."
5. Substitute low-calorie, low-fat foods whenever possible. Check caloric compositions on labels, because many products labeled "dietetic" contain the same number of calories as the original food products.
6. Keep low caloric foods in easy-to-open containers in the front of your refrigerator. Keep high-caloric foods in tightly sealed containers in the back of your refrigerator.
7. Throw away or alter your clothes as soon as they become too large. Don't give yourself "permission" to regain lost weight.
8. Know the caloric content of the alcohol you drink. The higher the proof, the higher the calories. **TIP:** Mixing drinks with club soda or dietetic ginger ale will cut down on the calories.
9. Shift your social life away from eating and drinking activities and towards physical activities, such as dancing or recreational sports.
10. Allow more time for meal preparation and enjoyment. Rushed meals contain "quickie" carbohydrates and "fast" fats.

Dr. DeBetz emphasizes, "FAT IS FAT! Remember—the sweeter the taste, the more bitter the aftertaste!"[93]

OSTEOPOROSIS

Symptoms

An estimated one out of every four women develops osteoporosis. This is a major, chronic disease involving an imbalance in the process by which bones are constantly broken down and rebuilt, a process known as bone remodeling. This process is carried out by bone cells called osteoclasts (which "resorb" or break down bone) and osteoblasts (which build bone). Osteoporosis develops when resorption exceeds formation, resulting in a loss of bone mass. DANGER: It is the principal underlying cause of bone fractures in older people, especially women. A fall, blow or lifting action can cause bones to break in someone with severe osteoporosis. It is the "silent disease" because it has no outward symptoms . . . until the bones become so weak that any sudden strain, bump or fall leads to a fracture. Often, the condition is first discovered on an X-ray taken for another purpose. Several non-invasive radiographic techniques are available to diagnose osteoporosis, including photon absorptiometry and computed tomography scanning. These are used to measure the bone mass of, for example, the spine, wrist or hip.

Natural Remedies

To protect against osteoporosis, your program calls for anti-resorptive remedies to inhibit the action of osteoclasts, stabilizing bone mass or increasing it modestly. The benefit is to reduce the likelihood of fractures.

Calcium Builds Strong Bones. "Your bones and teeth contain 99 percent of the calcium in your body. Since your body cannot make its own calcium, it depends on you to supply it. If you don't have enough of this mineral, your body takes the calcium it needs out of your bones and puts it into your blood so your body can continue to function. If—day after day, year after year—calcium is taken from your bones and not replaced via nutrition, your bones become weak and brittle . . . and break easily! This is both tragic and unnecessary—especially since it is so easy to get enough calcium in your diet," says Morris Notelovitz, M.D., Professor of Gynecology at the University of Florida, College of Medicine, in Gainesville.

Calcium Supplement. Dr. Notelovitz suggests a daily supplement of at least 1,000 milligrams of calcium. "It will help protect against depletion of vital calcium from your bones." He also suggests these natural remedies to help strengthen your skeleton and protect against "bone robbers":

Protein. More is not necessarily better. Protein increases calcium excretion more than it increases calcium absorption. "It would be wise to avoid an excess of protein or you will easily double or triple the rate of calcium—and therefore—bone loss!"

Exercise. You need it! "A sedentary lifestyle creates disuse osteoporosis. Clearly, you either use your bones or you lose them!" says Dr. Notelovitz. "Exercise is believed to be the only preventive or therapeutic measure that not only halts bone loss but actually stimulates the formation of new bone. Exercise increases blood flow to bones, bringing in bone-building nutrients." Recommended: at least 45 minutes of exercise daily!

Smoking. "Smoking will surely put you at a greater risk of osteoporosis because of an accelerated loss of bone. Give up this life-threatening habit. At the very least, cut down!" urges Dr. Notelovitz.

Soft Drinks. They can be bone robbers! "These drinks usually have a high rate of phosphorus which can displace the absorption of calcium so keep them out of your bone-building program."

Dr. Notelovitz also suggests improving your food program with more calcium from foods via low-fat or non-fat dairy products on a daily basis.[94]

How Good Is Your Calcium Supplement? There are over 30 supplements sold over-the-counter. But are these tablets really working? A study was conducted by Dr. Ralph Shangraw of the University of Maryland who tells us, "Of the various supplements, calcium carbonate is one of the least expensive forms available and you need fewer tablets to obtain equivalent amounts of calcium. *Note:* In order for calcium supplements to be absorbed by your body, they must first go through a dissolution process. Calcium carbonate has a higher dissolution rate." How can you tell if your supplement is working? Dr. Shangraw has an easy home test.

How To Test Your Calcium Supplement. Simply drop a single calcium carbonate tablet into six ounces of a 75 percent water and 25 percent vinegar solution, which mimics the acid environment of the stomach. Stir the mixture occasionally. After 30 minutes, a high-quality supplement should break up and be 75 percent dissolved. *Note:* Lack of disintegration is a clear indication of a calcium carbonate product with poor formulation. Try other products for a higher quality formulation.

Dr. Shangraw has found that factors such as meal size, timing of meals, protein intake, cooking methods, alcoholic beverages and dietary factor can affect absorption rates.[95]

Medications Can Interfere. Some medications, such as cortisone, antacids or laxatives, can interfere with your body's ability to absorb calcium. Ask your doctor if any medications you use will affect your bone health. If so, you may want to discuss calcium supplementation and an increase in calcium-rich foods.

❧ P ❧

PELVIC INFLAMMATORY DISEASE (PID)

Symptoms

Also known as *salpingitis*, this condition results from the spread of inflammation or infection within the fallopian tubes or ovaries. The organisms causing PID most often are transmitted sexually. It is a clinical syndrome in which an ascending microbial infection from the lower genital tract, usually the cervix, causes an inflammatory response in the fallopian tubes and adjacent structures. PID may expose the woman to serious long-term complications such as recurrent infections, chronic pelvic pain, ectopic pregnancy (occurring in the fallopian tube, which is unable to cope with the fetus as it expands and will cause pain and vaginal bleeding), and involuntary sterility. Be alert to lower abdominal pain which often increases with motion. Often, there may be mild pain that is dismissed as "just cramps." There may be fever, chills and a smelly vaginal discharge. Even walking may be profoundly painful. Chronic PID can develop with a continual low pelvic pain that is especially severe during intercourse.

CAUTION: Women who are sexually active at an early age, have multiple sex partners, engage in unprotected sexual activity, or use an intrauterine device (IUD) are at risk for PID. With a really bad infection, it can take as little as a few weeks to cause sterility!

Natural Remedies

Most doctors recommend that an intrauterine device used for birth control be removed from a woman who is diagnosed as having PID. It may be wise not to use the IUD. Many women with PID have sex partners who have no symptoms. Because of the risk of reinfection, however, sex partners should be treated. Even if they do not have symptoms, they may be infected with organisms that can cause PID.

Keep Yourself Clean. Since germs always present in the lower intestinal tract can cause infections in the genito-urinary system, the female, after a bowel movement, should wipe from front to back to avoid spreading infectious germs from rectum to vagina. *Remember*: PID occurs when disease-causing organisms travel upwards from the vagina and cervix into the reproductive organs, hence the importance of cleanliness, espe-

221

cially after a trip to the bathroom! And . . . medical supervision is mandatory.

POISON IVY

Symptoms

The old saying, "Leaflets three, let it be," can help you avoid poison ivy, poison oak, and poison sumac, all members of the plant genus *toxicodendron*; but these plants grow everywhere, in backyards as well as in woods and pastures. You are likely to develop symptoms if exposed to these plants, even by brief, accidental contact. Itching, redness, and blisters that burst and form weeping lesions are signs of allergy. Symptoms usually occur 24 to 48 hours after exposure, but may appear as long as 10 days later. The lesions are usually self-limited—they are at their worst after about five days and then improve in a week or two. The active oily ingredient common to all three plants is *urushiol*. This substance is easily transferred from one object to another—on clothes, tools, animal fur—and thus passed indirectly to people. CAREFUL: Because the urushiol is in the sap of the plant, rubbing or crushing the plant or leaf provides sufficient contact for an allergic reaction. DANGER: Smoke from burning plants may contain the urushiol on particles borne in the air and thus expose you to reactions on your skin or in your nose, throat, and lungs.

Natural Remedies

Several treatments are available. It is important to act promptly.

Quick Suds Remedy. Make sure your skin and clothes are free of all sap. Thorough sudsing of your skin or the use of 70 percent alcohol and rewashing of any clothing suspected of harboring urushiol should prevent spread of the lesions.

How to Relieve Inflammation. Wet cold compresses of water or boric acid will help relieve inflammation while the lesions are oozing.

Keep the Area Clean. Wash all exposed areas with water and soap or detergent. Be sure to clean thoroughly under your fingernails. The sap takes effect very quickly, so the washing must accompany promptly. If this is not possible, then plan to wash at the very earliest opportunity.

Take Repeat Showers. Lukewarm showers and cool or tepid compresses several times during the day between the repeat showers are very soothing.

Clean Contamination. Do not wear contaminated clothing until it is thoroughly washed. Do not wash it with other clothes. Take care to rinse thoroughly any implements used in washing. Automobile door handles or steering wheels may, after trips to the woods, cause poisoning among those who have not been near the plants. Decontaminate such articles by thorough washing in several changes of strong soap and water. (Dogs and cats may be decontaminated by washing; take care to avoid poisoning while washing the animal . . . and avoid a cat's outrage, too!)

Healing Tub Soak. Put a cup of cornstarch, oatmeal, or bicarbonate of soda in a tub of tepid water. Enjoy a 30 minute soak to help heal the symptoms. Repeat several times a day.

Calamine Lotion. A time-honored remedy, available at most pharmacies, it produces cooling and distracts your skin from the itching sensation. It also helps dry up the tiny blisters. Calamine lotion also leaves a powdery cover that absorbs the oozing, prompts a crust and keeps it from sticking to your garments. Apply calamine lotion several times a day. When the oozing stops, discontinue the remedy.

Water . . . but No Soap. You contract the rash and are in an area with water but no soap. What to do? Immediately wash with water. Do it thoroughly. Use your available canteen, hose or a moving stream. Water inactivates urushiol and is about as soothing as if soap were included.

Rubbing Alcohol. Wash your skin in lots and lots of rubbing alcohol to help remove the urushiol oil. Do **NOT** use a washcloth because it picks up this urushiol and spreads it around. Wash your hands after the alcohol rub . . . but rub *gently*, please.

Will Alcohol Prevent Poison Ivy? Definitely NOT!! Never apply alcohol before your venture into the wilds because it removes your protective skin oils and renders you all the more vulnerable to a poison ivy attack.

How You Can Prevent a Skin Outbreak. If you come in contact with any member of the poison ivy plant, immediately remove the oily resin (oleoresin) from your skin with soap and water. If this is done within 30 minutes, you are likely to prevent its development or at least reduce its severity. Wash your hands and under your fingernails. In the woods, the water of a running stream can be an effective cleanser and stop spreading of the oil.

To protect against poison ivy dermatitis, wear protective clothing when hiking or weeding: long sleeves, high socks and gloves; and then carefully remove the protective clothing and wash them in soap and water.

PREMENSTRUAL SYNDROME (PMS)

Symptoms

PMS is the term given to the group of physical and behavioral changes that often occur to women in the week before a menstrual period. These symptoms include distress, tension, abdominal bloating, fatigue, irritability or moodiness. There may be headache, backache, diarrhea, and nausea in more severe situations. Often, women may say or do things that alienate friends and family. Negative self-images may develop as some women try to cope with severe PMS symptoms. Because of fluid retention, there are feelings of bloating, with swelling in the ankles, abdomen, and breasts.

Natural Remedies

To gain better control over this monthly situation, nutritional programs are often the foundation.

Important Vitamins to Ease PMS. Patricia Allen, M.D., Clinical Instructor of Obstetrics and Gynecology at the College of Physicians and Surgeons, Columbia University, in New York City, pinpoints two important vitamins:

Vitamin A. "It has a mild diuretic effect and so may partly relieve swelling of the breasts and lower abdomen. It is also an immune system strengthener that may help ward off stress and fatigue." Dr. Allen lists these rich food sources of vitamin A: golden-fleshed fruits and vegetables, especially squash, yams, carrots, peaches, nectarines, apricots.

Vitamin B_6 (Pyridoxine). It is a key brain-cell nutrient and is needed to help balance certain brain chemical functions to protect against the moodiness of PMS. "Some physicians recommend taking the vitamin at least three days before expected symptoms and continuing until three days into the menstrual period—typically starting with 50 milligrams a day and increasing this up to 200 milligrams until you notice results. At higher dosages, you may risk some mild gastric acidity, the only worrisome possible side effect. TIP: Pyridoxine should be taken in its B-complex form, not alone, because in high doses it tends to deplete the other B vitamins in the body." Dr. Allen lists these natural sources of Vitamin B_6: whole grain breads and cereals, cabbage, fresh vegetables, brown rice, Brewer's yeast, milk and eggs.

Minerals Are Soothing. Dr. Patricia Allen notes that women with PMS also are subjected to stress and this can be soothed with minerals. "A calcium shortage can show up as weakness and depression or excitability and anxiety." She also recommends magnesium and potassium. "In one nutritional study, women with PMS showed a lower magnesium level between body cells than women who were symptom-free. Potassium, too, is particularly essential to the control of PMS as levels of this mineral decline when sodium and water are retained premenstrually." Dr. Allen lists these natural sources of calcium, magnesium and potassium: low-fat dairy products, low-sodium cheeses, dark green and yellow vegetables, such as broccoli, asparagus, squash and zucchini. "Vegetables should be raw or minimally cooked, with little water, preferably steamed or stir-fried." Also include whole grain breads and cereals, bananas, oranges, tomatoes, apricots, and fresh fruit or vegetable juices.[96]

Keep Yourself Active. Sustained, vigorous exercise—the kind that gets your pulse rate up and keeps it there is very beneficial as a natural antidote to PMS. Try swimming, cycling, jogging, skipping rope, aerobic dancing. Physical activity helps decrease fluid and sodium retention and tones up a sluggish digestive tract and your abdominal muscles.

The Plant that Eases Pain. The oil from the evening primrose flower is rich in linoleic acid, one of the body's essential fatty acids and the basis of prostaglandins—hormone-like substances produced by the body's tissues. There are different kinds of prostaglandins, though. PGE_1 is suspected of having a role in PMS. A woman who takes an evening primrose capsule provides her body with linoleic acid for the increase of PGE_1 prostaglandin. A steady production of PGE_1, which can be maintained with the linoleic acid of the evening primrose oil, may suppress PMS symptoms. Evening primrose oil is available in capsule form at health stores and pharmacies, too.

Control Intake of Salt, Sugar, Caffeine. Niels H. Lauersen, M.D., Professor of Obstetrics and Gynecology at Mt. Sinai Hospital, in New York City, suggests much less intake of salt (to avoid edema or water buildup). Avoid refined carbohydrates such as sugar because "it will go right into the bloodstream, cause low-blood sugar attacks and will lead to headaches, depression, agitation and irritability." Best to emphasize complex or natural carbohydrates instead of refined foods. Caffeine is found in coffee, tea, cola and chocolate drinks. "Caffeine stimulates the brain, which in turn affects the central nervous system, and the activity of the heart and circulatory system. Many women find that caffeine tends to worsen PMS symptoms in general. The woman would be wise to switch to decaffeinated coffee, caffeine-free teas, and no-caffeine carbonated beverages during her cycle."[97]

Keep Yourself Warm. A warm bath increases blood flow and relaxes cramped and congested pelvic muscles. Add one cup of sea salt and one cup of baking soda to a warm tub and enjoy a 30-minute soak. *Alternative*: Drink lots of hot herbal teas or natural beverages. Apply a heating pad or hot water bottle on your stomach for five minutes at a time. Very soothing.

CASE HISTORY—*Conquers "The Curse" with Natural Remedies*

She was so fearful of her monthly "curse" as she called it, Annette K. N. would develop symptoms before the actual onset of PMS. She tried medications, but they had side effects, itching and a sleepy feeling. As a sales supervisor, when she fell asleep behind the wheel while on business trips, she realized she needed to find a safer way to cope with her symptoms. She contacted a female OB/GYN physician who said that she, herself, eased distress by taking vitamins A and B_6, as well as minerals (described earlier). She also eliminated salt, sugar, and caffeine. But for severe symptoms, she would take several capsules of evening primrose oil as a "natural medicine." She told Annette K. N. to do the same. It worked wonders! Her symptoms so subsided, she no longer felt "enslaved" to her "curse" and was now a "free woman!"

PROSTATE GLAND

Symptoms

The prostate rests just below the bladder and completely surrounds the urethra, the tube that carries urine and semen through the penis and out of the body. Its main function is to supply most of the lubricating fluid that transports sperm cells during ejaculation. The size of a nickel (in diameter), the prostate may cause serious trouble, especially in men over age 50. A major disorder is prostatitis or inflammation. Warning symptoms include one or more of the following: lower back pain, fever, pain on urination, and pain under the scrotum, and pain in the pelvis. Illness may range from simple inflammation to life-threatening cancer. CAUTION: Prostate cancer frequently develops with few warning signs. They may include weak or interrupted flow of urine; inability to urinate or difficulty in beginning to urinate; more noticeable could be the need to urinate frequently, especially at night. It is essential to bring symptoms to the attention of your health practitioner as early as possible to help protect against worsening of any condition.

Natural Remedies

Help your prostate function with youthful vigor with some reported programs.

Slant Board Technique. A San Diego, California physician was diagnosed by other doctors as having chronic non-bacterial prostatitis. (This type usually starts as a urinary tract infection and then spreads to the prostate.) Jay Cohen, M.D. tells of being plagued by symptoms for five years, which ranged from lower back pain, muscular soreness, and aching in the area below the genitals to occasional painful urination. "Most distressing was a constant pain on both sides of my groin, which progressed to a swollen and tender epididymis (sperm storage sites in the scrotum), and a pain so intense, it severely limited my activities." Dr. Cohen tried a variety of treatments prescribed by three different urologists with modest help. He was about to take an antibiotic (carbenicillin) when "something surprising" occurred to provide a natural remedy.

"Having noticed that my epididymis swelled and ached the more I was on my feet, I thought I would try using my wife's slant board, which raises the feet above the head at an angle of 30 degrees. Understand, I always laughed at my wife for her unconventional ideas. I felt quite strange the first time I found myself looking up at my toes. But my embarrassment faded as my symptoms gradually but steadily disappeared. Now, over a year later, I am virtually free of symptoms. I am far better than when I was taking the antibiotics. A long day will still evoke some tenderness and swelling, but it disappears quickly once I am back on the slant board."

Slant Board Heals Prostate Disorder. Dr. Cohen says he uses the slant board for 20 minutes, three times a day. He is free of all medication and "fully active"—swimming, windsurfing, and sitting without discomfort. *Benefit*: The tilted position may enhance the drainage of secretions and swelling, similar to the effect of elevating swollen feet. *Note*: If you have cardiovascular distress, high blood pressure, intracranial conditions, glaucoma, vascular fragility or breathing disorders, Dr. Cohen suggests caution as well as approval by your health practitioner.[98]

Stress, Personality Problems, Smoking, Spicy Foods. You may well abuse your prostate (as well as other parts of your body) with stress. Many symptoms of prostatitis are related to muscle stress. It happens because stress causes an increase in the tone of the urethral sphincter muscle. Donald H. Rudnick, M.D., of Pomona, California links stress to prostatitis. "In my practice, where 'prostatitis' comprises 15 percent of patient visits, the one common thread binding all patients together is chronic, unrelenting stress. The stress may result from problems in any of life's spheres—work, education or family. The various constitutional symptoms from the (prostatitis) disease respond best when patients are removed from their source of stress—at vacation time, when the big job is finally done, or when the family dispute is settled.

"Furthermore," notes Dr. Rudnick, "prostatitis patients are invariably heavy smokers, heavy caffeine partakers, and spicy food eaters. These substances are known as urothelial irritations. Elimination of them from the diet always prompts symptomatic improvement.

"I have always felt that prostatitis is a disease of the person and not simply an inflammation of the prostate and have, therefore, given advice regarding both dietary and physical and mental hygiene along with antibiotic therapy to more effectively eliminate the chances of relapse or recurrence."[99]

Limit Animal Fat Intake. In some studies, it was shown that heavy intake of animal food products could predispose to cancer of the prostate much more than those who limited such foods. The body uses animal fat to make excess sex hormones. A runaway supply may cause distress in the prostate, hence the need to control the production of hormones. This can be done by limiting intake of animal foods and following a low-fat food program.

Nutritional Remedies. Increase intake of beta-carotene foods to prevent formation of hurtful free radicals that can cause prostate cancer and other disorders. Include cruciferous vegetables (Brussels sprouts, broccoli, carrots, cauliflower, cabbage). Boost intake of vitamin C and vitamin E, which help block production of threatening and cancer-causing free radicals in cells. Selenium and zinc, which are also necessary, are available from wheat germ, bran, tuna fish, onions, tomatoes, and broccoli.

The Zinc Connection. In some situations, zinc may help reduce swelling of the prostate gland. The prostate uses much zinc and is a deposition site for body zinc stores. It has been helpful in supplements of 150 milligrams daily over a period of two to four months to ease inflammation and swelling.

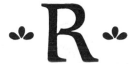

RASHES

Symptoms

Several or clusters of dots that may appear anywhere on the body. Colors range from white to different shades of red, black and blue. They may erupt as bumps and even break out in blisters. Some go away, others become an unsightly and stubborn plague. Itching is often an annoying symptom.

Natural Remedies

Heat and moisture aggravate rashes and allow microorganisms to invade, producing a secondary infection. An important natural remedy is to keep your skin cool and dry. Light, loose-fitting clothes, air-conditioning or fans, cool showers followed by the use of dusting powder, and limiting physical activity are helpful.

Prickly Heat. Also called miliaria, it is caused by temporary blockage of the sweat duct openings on the skin surface. Most common in areas where skin surfaces are close together; in skin folds, for example, and overweight conditions. Gently bathe in plain water, or water plus a mild soap.

Quick Cooling Remedy. Spread a cornstarch and water paste over the affected area and let remain for several hours. Then splash off (gently, please) with cool water. Repeat twice a day.

Cool Off that Rash. Once a heat rash develops, a light sprinkling of talcum powder or cornstarch will usually bring some relief. Try cool baths with a cup of colloidal oatmeal (available in pharmacies) added to the water. Or else, combine one cup of oatmeal with two cups of laundry starch in the water, and soak in the cool tub.

Chafed Skin. A rash breaks out when your skin is rubbed raw by repeated friction with an opposing skin surface, like the inner thighs, or irritation from rough clothing, like the seam in a shirt. Avoid heavy-duty fabrics. Try not to exercise in hot, humid weather. Avoid using any greasy ointments or products containing local anesthetics such as benzocaine, which can intensify allergic reactions. Clothes should be cool and comfortable.

You may also have an allergic reaction to detergents used in washing clothes (and yourself, too.) If you see an outbreak after such products, discontinue them and seek other brands. *Note*: Many rashes are allergic reactions to the perfumed fabric softener pads that are placed in clothes dryers.

Hints, Tips, Suggestions. Keep cool and dry by wearing clothes made of natural fibers such as cotton or linen. Avoid any tight-fitting garments which trap moisture, especially those made of rubber or polyester. Pat yourself thoroughly dry after bathing; apply calamine lotion to the rash and allow it to dry. Dust yourself with a cornstarch-based body powder before getting dressed. Be alert to certain products that contain irritating chemicals, including cosmetics, cleaning agents, or those you come in contact with at work.

RAYNAUD'S SYNDROME

Symptoms

Cold hands, especially during the winter, becomes annoyingly uncomfortable for those who have this disorder. It is named after Maurice Raynaud, a French physician, who first described the condition in 1862. It involves more than chilly fingertips. Raynaud's often also affects the toes, sometimes the nose and ears as well. It is not always a cold weather complaint. A cool breeze on a hot day may bring on an attack. The ice-cold feeling in the extremities may be triggered by drafty rooms, vibrating tools, or emotional stress. Raynaud's is seen among those who work with their hands—computer operators, typists, meat cutters, musicians (especially pianists and guitarists), and those who use such vibrating tools as chain saws and jackhammers. The problem may be traced to using the palm of the hand as a hammer, even from only one episode. CAREFUL: Chronic exposure to the cold, repeated exposure to alternating hot and cold temperature, or a case of frostbite may lead to vulnerability to Raynaud's. Other culprits may be drugs, such as nicotine, oral contraceptives, ergot-containing medications used to treat migraine headaches, or beta-blockers that treat high blood pressure all may cause problems. *Note*: In most patients, the problem is one of a localized over-sensitivity to hormones that cause blood vessels to constrict.

Natural Remedies

John A. Mills, M.D., Director of the Massachusetts General Hospital Arthritis Clinic, in Boston, who treats many Raynaud patients, has one clue to this disorder.

Emotional Upset. "Emotional disturbances alone can alter blood flow. People sometimes get cold hands when they are anxious or hot hands when they are stressed. I've asked patients whether they have been stricken with Raynaud's while emotionally upset. Perhaps one in six or eight patients has told me, 'Yes, that will do it.' Others attribute their attacks entirely to the cold." TIP: If you experience icy cold hands and feet after an emotional upset . . . control yourself and protect your emotions against such situations.

To help protect yourself against an attack, Dr. John A. Mills recommends these basic precautions:

- Before driving to work in the morning, start your car, turn on your heater, then go back into the house for several minutes while your vehicle warms up.
- If possible, arrange for parking close to your place of employment.
- Keep your head covered while outdoors so your body is forced to expel heat through your other extremities.
- If your hands become chilled and you cannot get indoors, try to promote circulation by swimming your arms in a perpendicular fashion with your fingers outstretched.
- Wear enough extra clothing, even when indoors, to create the feeling that you would like to take something off.

"Wearing gloves, a hat and other extra clothing can help to forestall a Raynaud's attack. But ignoring the problem and permitting frequent and long-lasting episodes can result in ulcers forming on the fingertips. If they become infected, gangrene might follow so do not disregard this situation. Feeling just a little warmer than you would otherwise like to be helps to induce maximum circulation in your hands and feet," adds Dr. Mills.[100]

Hints, Tips, Suggestions. To help keep your hands and body warm, try these helpful remedies:

- If you smoke, stop. Nicotine narrows blood vessels.
- Protect your hands by wearing thermal gloves under windproof

mittens. Warm your feet with good socks under thermally lined boots. You may place a reflective innersole in your shoes.

- Try not to touch cold metal with your bare hands. Cover outside door knobs and keys with rubber caps. Cover your auto's steering wheel with insulated leather or sheepskin. If your seat cover is plastic or leather, sit on a fabric cushion.
- Wash produce in lukewarm water.
- Keep wrists and neck warmly covered. Nerves in your neck influence the blood vessels in your hands; if these neck nerves are chilled, they cause a tightening of hand vessels.
- Are you taking drugs that interfere with blood flow? Check it out with your doctor.
- Use a holder or several napkins when handling cold beverage containers.
- Dehydration can bring on chills by reducing your blood volume. Protect against the big chill by drinking lots of fluids such as caffeine-free beverages, hot cider, salt-free broth.

CAREFUL: Caffeine constricts blood vessels, so avoid such products as coffee, chocolate, many soft drinks, and commercial tea.

RESPIRATORY TRACT

Symptoms

Chilliness, back and muscle pain, sore throat, annoying cough, difficulty in getting enough air during physical activities, susceptibility to various inhaled infections, poor skin pallor.

Natural Remedies

You need to improve your breathing! Dr. Jack Soltanoff, Chiropractor-Nutritionist, from West Hurley, New York, explains, "Breathing is something we all take for granted. You can be eating the best organically grown food in the world in correct combinations, but if your breathing is shallow and constricted, you're not utilizing all that good food properly. You're not getting full benefit from it."

Improve Your Posture. Dr. Soltanoff notes, "Poor breathing is usually linked to poor posture. When you're not standing straight, your lungs cannot fill up properly. Exercise will improve both posture and the accessory breathing muscles. Better breathing will then become automatic. If you find you are not breathing properly, then exercise regularly. Even if you are breathing properly, you will still benefit from specific breathing exercises." *Examples:*

Morning Respiratory Rejuvenator. Lie flat on your back. Place a small rolled towel or pillow between your shoulder blades. Do not put a pillow beneath your head. Keep knees bent. Lift arms slowly up and backward overhead while you breathe in through your nose for the slow count of five. Slowly lower arms to your sides while you exhale forcibly through your mouth for a count of five. Exhale thoroughly.

Breathe In . . . and Out . . . As Often As Possible. This is very helpful when in the open or while taking a brisk walk. Fill your lungs to the maximum as often as possible. Breathe in through your nose. Feel that expansion in your abdominal region as it gradually goes up to your chest. Fill your lungs with fresh air. Hold it for a moment. Try a bit more. Okay . . . now fully exhale through your mouth. Repeat frequently . . . but if you feel tired, hold off.

Seated Respiratory Exercise. Sit on a firm chair. Breathe in *slowly* through your nose. Fill your lungs. Then exhale slowly with your lips pressed close to your teeth, while keeping a narrow slit open between them. Force out the air in short, detached breaths through this narrow slit. You should feel much invigoration via your abdominal, diaphragm and rib muscles because you are forcing air through this small opening. Repeat five times.

Dr. Soltanoff recommends, "Much walking but do it briskly to get your lungs working, your heart pumping and your cells and tissues oxygenated and cleansed. Walk regularly. Start with half a mile to one mile. Gradually increase both pace and distance until you cover a mile in about twenty minutes. Six miles a day is ideal, but only if you can do so comfortably. **TIP:** Aim for one hour of brisk walking daily and your respiratory system will thank you for the rest of your life."[101]

Get Into the Better Breathing Habit. Start your day off with deep breathing. Every morning on arising, walk around your bedroom on your tiptoes with your hands reaching high over your head and your diaphragm raised as high as your strength will allow you to lift it. Easy to do—just draw in a good, full, deep breath and raise your chest as high as possible. Make this a morning exercise . . . every morning, please!

Pure Air Is Your Invisible Food. Refresh your respiratory system by flushing out toxic wastes and then breathing in cleansing air. Detoxify your respiratory system and enjoy a healthier oxygen-nourished body and mind, too!

⁂ S ⁂

SHINGLES

Symptoms

Also known as herpes zoster, shingles is a painful viral disease. It is caused by the varicella-zoster virus, the same virus responsible for chickenpox. After a bout of the disease, the virus retreats to sensory nerve cells, eventually hiding around the spine in one or several groups of nerve cells called ganglia, where it lies dormant. In some people, the virus becomes active again when the immune system becomes weakened, whether by age, another illness, emotional stress or physical trauma. Early symptoms include pain, or an abnormal sensation in a major nerve; fever, headache, nausea or malaise. Within days, the skin near the affected nerve develops a band or belt of blisters. A rash follows, usually on one side of the body. The term "shingles" means *belt* in Latin, because the ailment often appears in a band-like pattern on the skin. The pain is described as continuous aching, itching or burning, often with severe shooting pains triggered by touching or moving the affected area. People who endure long-term pain may also experience depression, insomnia, and weight loss, which adds psychological suffering to the physical pain. *Note*: The virus should not be confused with the herpes simplex viruses of cold sore and genital sore discomfort. Unlike them, the shingles virus is not related to any kind of sexual activity. Rather, the culprit is the chickenpox virus that lies in wait until the immune system is weakened and then it strikes with a vengeance.

Natural Remedies

At the beginning stages of shingles, give a boost to your immune system to help counteract the reaction.

Nutrients for Stronger Immune System. A vitamin B complex supplement helps to rebuild and regenerate the nerve cells that are hurt by the virus. Vitamin C, in doses up to 1,000 milligrams daily will help improve the cells and tissues of the skin and nourish the aching collagen and nerve cells, too. In combination, these vitamins help strengthen the immune system to ease shingles outbreaks and hurt.

237

Lysine: The Amino Acid that Heals Shingles. In reported treatments, lysine, an amino acid, helped over eight out of every ten herpes patients tested. Dosages given were about 1,000 milligrams daily. Lysine is found in grains, but much is lost during the refining, baking, and even the toasting of bread. It is available in supplements. Researchers feel that lysine taken at the onset of shingles is most beneficial, although it is useful at any stage of the ailment. Lysine helps ease pain and inhibits the spread of the herpes virus.[102]

Calamine Lotion Is Soothing. You may make this yourself, or ask your neighborhood pharmacist to prepare the lotion. Add to calamine lotion, 20 percent isopropyl alcohol and one percent of phenol, and one percent of menthol. (If the phenol is too strong or the menthol too cool, dilute the liniment with equal parts of water.) Apply this Calamine Lotion frequently to the shingles blisters. When they are dried and scabbed over, discontinue use. Start a lotion that has both phenol and menthol. Your pharmacist has such a product.

Keep the Area Cool. Dip a clean hand towel or wash cloth in cold water. Squeeze it out. Apply gently to the affected area. It is as soothing as ice on a burn. *Never* use heat, which will further injure your blistered skin.

Soak in a Cornstarch Bath. If your outbreak is below the neck, treat yourself to a soothing bath. Add one cup of cornstarch or colloidal oatmeal (from any pharmacy) to one tub of comfortably cool water. Be careful as you get into the tub. Give yourself a 30-minute soak to calm the pain. Especially beneficial before bedtime to help you sleep well.

When Blisters Are Gone . . . but Pain Remains. Cool off with ice. Place some cubes in a plastic bag and stroke the painful skin. This "confuses" the nerves and tends to ease the pain.

---------------------------- ❧ ----------------------------

CASE HISTORY—*Nips Shingles Nerve Damage Before It Could Spread*

At the very first signs of the cluster of blisters on his shoulders, Joseph DiG. sought help from an internist. Immediately, he was put on a nutritional program with emphasis upon vitamin B complex, vitamin C (1,000 milligrams daily), and lysine (1,000 milligrams daily). The internist told Joseph DiG. that the nutrients would slow reproduction of the varicella zoster virus and shorten the course of infection. Together with cool applications and a twice-a-day cornstarch soak, Joseph DiG. was able to nip the shingles attack before it could spread. Placed on a stress-reduction program, his immune system was strengthened, and he was soon healed of this threat to his nerve system.

SINUS DISORDERS

Symptoms

Sinuses are hollow air spaces located within the skull or bones of the head surrounding the nose. Anything that causes a swelling in the nose—be it a viral or bacterial infection or an allergic reaction—can similarly affect the sinuses. Headache upon awakening in the morning is characteristic of a sinus disorder. An inflammation inside the nose because of a lingering cold or allergy attack will cause nasal passages to swell and chronically block or inhibit the natural flow of mucus. Congestion could lead to a bacterial infection that is responsible for staphylococcus and streptococcus infections and some forms of pneumonia. The very early symptoms are those of a lingering cold; be alert to extreme fatigue, high fever, stubborn headaches, facial pain, or a feeling of overall achiness.

Natural Remedies

To build resistance to sinus disorders, strengthen your immune system with improved living methods, such as:

- Appropriate amounts of rest, a well-balanced diet and exercise help you function at an efficient level and maintain a general resistance to infections.
- You may find partial relief from sinusitis when humidifiers are installed in your home, particularly when the room air is heated by a dry forced-air system. Air conditioners help to provide an even temperature. Electrostatic filters—attached to heating and air conditioning equipment—are valuable in removing irritants from the air.
- Cigarette smoke and other air pollutants should be avoided. Allergic inflammation in the nose will predispose you to a strong reaction to all irritants. CAUTION: Curtail alcohol because it causes a swelling of the nasal-sinus membranes.
- You may be uncomfortable in swimming pools treated with chlorine,

since this substance is irritating to the lining of the nose and sinuses. Divers often experience congestion and infection when water is forced into the sinuses from the nasal passages.

- Air travel may be a problem. A bubble of air trapped within your body expands as air pressure in a plane is reduced. This expansion causes pressure in surrounding tissues and can result in a blockage of the sinuses or eustachian tubes. The result may be extreme discomfort in the sinuses or middle ear during the plane's ascent or descent.

- Discomfort often can be lessened by inhaling steam from a vaporizer or tea kettle. A hot water bottle; hot, wet compresses; an electric heating pad applied over the inflamed area may prove to be soothing.

- Sleep with your window open to allow fresh air and some humidity to circulate in your room. This keeps your nasal passages from swelling.

- During the day, at home or at work, be sure to have adequate ventilation. You need to boost humidity levels. **CAREFUL:** If you work near copy machines or other office equipment that give off vapors, be sure to have open windows nearby or you may inflame your nasal passages.

- To help release blockages, take frequent steamy showers. Humidity helps keep your cilia (nasal hairs) working and your sinuses drained.

Take a Steam Break. Several times a day, lean over a pan full of steaming water. Drape a towel over your head to create a tent. Breathe in the vapors as they float up toward your nostrils. Do this several times and you will help keep your sinuses in good condition.

Lots of Liquids. Comfortably hot herbal teas, salt-free broths, coffee substitutes, soups will help keep your body lubricated and your sinuses well humidified. You need this extra moisture to keep mucus moving. Drink these liquids throughout the day.

How to Spice Your Sinuses for Better Breathing. Several spices that you eat will help you breathe better. These include garlic (it contains ingredients that act much like a chemical in loosening congestion), horseradish (acts like a natural decongestant so you have healthier sinuses), and Cajun spice (especially cayenne peppers, those little red torches that contain capsaicin, which revives your nerve fibers and functions as a natural nasal decongestant). *How to Use:* Spice up your foods with any of these items—a little bit goes a long way. They make your eyes water and your nose run and clear away sinus blockage! Use in place of salt or pepper.

Quick Pain Healer. Apply a warm washcloth dipped in comfortably hot water to the area over your cheekbones and bridge of your nose. Let it remain about five minutes and the pain will subside. Repeat as often as necessary.

SKIN

Symptoms

Blemishes, discoloration, swelling, fragility, and breakouts are only some of the reactions that indicate your skin has problems. The quality of your skin is a reflection of your general health. Truly good looking skin exudes a picture of youth . . . at any age. You can have "forever young" skin with better self-care and prompt attention to any symptoms.

Natural Remedies

Here are programs to help improve your skin and overcome common and uncommon disorders.

Blackheads or Whiteheads. Keep away from whatever blocks the pores. This includes greases, oils or creams you put on your skin. Switch to a water-based product. Keep out of the sun. It will redden and swell your skin, which further blocks your pores. Do not rub your skin. Wash and dry your skin gently. Do not squeeze blackheads! You may injure the follicular wall and cause the contents to break through the wall of the follicle into the surrounding tissue, where it will produce inflammation. Your dermatologist can either extract the blackheads or show you the proper technique for removing them yourself.

Bruises. Apply ice as soon as possible after injury to tighten the capillaries, slow the bleeding and swelling. Keep the area elevated, if possible. Recurring bruises could be a deficiency of such nutrients as riboflavin, folic acid, bioflavonoids, or vitamin C.

Cracks. They often appear on the backs of your hands and around your knuckles and fingers. Cracked skin invites bacterial infection so take quick action. Soak your hands in cool water. Dry gently. Apply ordinary petroleum jelly. Do this *gently*. Put on clean cotton gloves to be worn during the day. Or, do this every night before retiring and let the moisture soak in.

Dry Skin. The cause is lack of water—not oil—in the thin top layer of your skin. Limit bathing or showering and use either mild or a superfatted soap (or no soap at all) in those dry areas. After bathing, pat yourself dry gently and apply a moisturizer. It locks in water that was absorbed into your skin while bathing. Apply this moisturizer *promptly* after the bath. You may also apply a dab of any vegetable oil or even hydrogenated cooking products (such as Crisco) onto the dry area. They are excellent skin lubricants, safe and pure. And . . . raise humidity levels in your home. Add moisture by placing water-filled pans on your radiators. Moisture from houseplants will evaporate into the air to boost humidity.

Bumps, Lumps. Apply a comfortably hot, wet compress every few hours to ease pain and accelerate healing. Do **not** squeeze bumps because this may spread the infection. You could prevent more bumps by taking a shower with an antibacterial soap twice a day.

Oily Skin. Soap and water is the most efficient way of minimizing the degree of oiliness. Cleansing creams or lotions worsen the problem. If you must use a cleansing cream to remove makeup, follow it up with soap and water. If washing is inconvenient, at work or school, then premoistened cleansing pads can be used. Another way to remove excess oils is to blot with special absorbent papers, which are available at pharmacies and cosmetic counters. Wear waterbased makeup rather than cream or oil-based products. For some, a bit of alcohol on a cloth is helpful since it will dissolve the oil.

Feed Yourself A Healthy Skin

To look your best, feed your skin with an optimal amount of the needed raw materials (i.e., nutrients). These include:

Fats —preferably from plant foods and seafoods. Your skin needs essential fatty acids to help protect it against eruptions and premature aging. A small amount goes a long way.

Zinc —stimulates antibody production for protecting against invading organisms that threaten your skin.

Vitamin A —preferably beta-carotene from plant sources, to maintain a healthy skin.

Vitamin B complex —emphasis upon thiamine, riboflavin, and biotin, as well as the others that help nourish the cells and tissues.

Vitamin C —maintains the connective tissue to give your body a smooth resilience. Builds collagen to support your structure.

Vitamin E —promotes manufacture of glutathione peroxidase (GSH), which protects hormones that influence skin health.

Selenium —a lesser known but vital mineral needed to keep skin moisturized and youthful.

Zinc —encourages youthful metabolism, which is a major function of daily skin growth and repair.

Water —a minimum of six cups of fresh water daily keeps skin moisturized, cleansed, younger and smoother. Perhaps the most vital nutrient your skin will ever need!

SORE THROAT

Symptoms

Recurring coughs, choking, hoarseness, soreness, all give you a sore throat. Never neglect any persistent symptom that refuses to go away, since it is your body's way of telling you that something is wrong and has to be corrected.

Natural Remedies

Soothe your throat with these helps.

Throat Tickle. It may be bitter tasting, but it does ease that tickle: suck on a whole clove (the kind you stick into a baked meat roast). Works in minutes.

Sore Throat. Gargle with warm salt water. The high salt concentration tends to work with an appreciable antibacterial action. Saline reduces swelling of the tissues.

Keep Your Mouth Closed. During breathing, that is. Instead, use your nose for breathing to deflect irritating airstreams from your throat.

Hoarseness. Breathe moisturized-air. With either a vaporizer or humidifier turned on, breathe slowly and deeply for fifteen minutes to relieve hoarseness.

Sensitive Throat. Apply a comfortably hot pack against the front of your throat, in the hollow, for about 15 minutes. Repeat five to seven times a day. Helps ease hoarseness.

"Swelling" in Throat. Wastes trapped in the uvula, an area in the throat, give a feeling of swelling. Something is trapped. To dislodge a trapped particle, sip ice water to reduce the swelling and promote cleansing.

Back of Throat Parchedness. Add two tablespoons of salt to one quart of warm water. Pour a small amount into your hand. Slowly inhale through your nose. Or . . . use an eyedropper to squirt the solution into your nose. It helps offset that parched feeling.

If You Smoke—STOP! Smoking irritates and inflames the nasopharynx, depletes vitamin C, paralyzes the respiratory cilia, which move wastes out of the infected area. Smoking is ruinous to your throat . . . and the rest of your body, too!

Lots of Warm Liquids . . . Every Two Hours. For a persistent sore throat, comfortably hot liquids are very soothing. Best not to drink cold beverages, since they impede the movement of wastes and cause congestion. Plan to sip hot liquids throughout the day, if possible, to heal your sore throat.

Dry Cough. Use a vaporizer and take comfortably warm showers. **CAREFUL:** If any dry cough is accompanied by chills, fever, chest pain, wheezing, shortness of breath, or if it brings up a discolored sputum, seek medical help promptly. It could be pneumonia!

Refresh with Liquids. A dry, grating throat is parched for liquids. Plain water is excellent because it helps hydrate your sandy throat in a matter of minutes. Plan to drink lots of liquids throughout the day. **AVOID:** Milk drinks which coat your throat and produce mucus to further irritate tissues; citrus juices may burn an already hurting throat; caffeine-containing beverages have a counterproductive diuretic reaction that will further dehydrate your body.

Correct Your Sleeping Posture. Recurring sore throat may be traced to (1) sleeping with one's mouth open which dries out the pharygeal tissues and (2) sleeping with one's head too low, which may send a backup of stomach acids into the throat during the night. Such acids irritate delicate tissues. **TIP:** Tilt your bed frame so your head is about five inches higher than the foot. Use bricks for a steady hold. **CAREFUL:**

Do not add pillows under your head since they will force you to bend in the waistline, adding unnecessary pressure to your esophagus to worsen the condition. Avoid food or drink three hours before retiring, and . . . keep your mouth closed while sleeping!

Try a Facial Sauna. Inhale steam for fifteen minutes and moisturize your dry throat. A salt-based inhalation moistens your nasal passages and increases throat humidity. It is considered a natural decongestant nasal spray.

STIFF NECK

Symptoms

A painful stiffness when you try to turn your head in any direction. Bending is hurtful. Muscular aches and stiffness along the nape of your neck, extending down across your shoulders, sometimes lower. In extreme situations, you can hardly move your neck because it feels imprisoned in a vise.

Natural Remedies

Your neck muscles stiffen if you keep your head in an unnatural position. DANGER: Do not hold your head pushed forward, with your ears in front of your shoulders. An occupational hazard is one that calls for a bent-over position for hours at a time. Your first remedy: keep your head up! Never remain in any position too long.

Neck flexibility is something you never think about until you start to back your automobile. Your neck hurts when you try to turn! You can maintain and even increase neck flexibility with proper exercise.

According to Dennis Humphrey, EdD, professor in the Biomedical Services Department at Southwest Missouri State University, Springfield, not all commonly used exercises are safe. He outlines several simple remedies. But first . . .

How to Begin. Warm up your body first, with 10 to 15 minutes of walking, jogging or other aerobic activity.

How to Do Exercises. Each one is to be done five times. "Use slow, smooth motions. Stretch to the point of slight discomfort. Hold for a count of 10," says Dr. Humphrey. "Avoid any bouncing motion.

As flexibility increases, hold the stretch for a count of 20 to 30, doing them 10 times each."

1. Drop your chin to your chest and hold that position. *Benefit*: Stretches the back of your neck.
2. Turn your head to the left. Hold it. Then turn your head to the right. Hold it. *Benefit*: Stretches the muscles in the front of your neck.
3. Lean your head to the right, as if trying to place your right ear on your right shoulder and hold it; then repeat to the other side. (Don't raise shoulders in this exercise.) *Benefit*: stretches the muscles in the sides of your neck.

CAUTION: Dr. Humphrey says there are two common neck exercises that he does not recommend "because they may cause nerve-root compression in the neck, particularly if there is some degenerative disk or joint disease. Two exercises to avoid are: (1) hyperextending your neck (looking up toward the ceiling) and (2) neck circles (rolling your head around in a circular fashion)."[103]

Ice-Heat Remedy. An ice pack on the back of your neck will help suppress any potential swelling or stiffness. After the ice has cooled the inflammation, apply heat, whether from a hot shower or a heating pad.

Seven Remedies to Ease Stiff Neck Pain. The California Medical Association explains, "If your work requires you to remain with your head in one position for prolonged periods of time, you are susceptible to neck strain." The Association offers these seven remedies to prevent and ease this discomfort:

1. Try not to sit in any one position too long. Specifically, do not keep your head bent over reading or sewing, or fixed on the television or computer screen without intervals of relaxation. In most jobs, it is possible to change positions, get up and stretch, or do a few simple neck-resting exercises from time to time. This not only relaxes your muscles but also relieves tension which, of itself, tightens up your neck muscles and gives you pain.
2. While driving, your seat should be at the right height so you can look over the steering wheel without straining. Your seat should be forward enough so you don't have to flex your neck forward. All cars have a head rest (or have one installed!) so your neck cannot get thrown backwards into an extended position.
3. Sit on a straight-backed chair. Sit up straight and keep your neck straight.

4. Don't try to compensate for your height at the expense of neck comfort. If you're short, don't thrust your chin upward. If you're tall, don't slump. Either habit places a strain on your neck. **TIP:** Use a sideways motion when getting up or lying down, instead of sitting up head-first or lying down backward from a sitting position.

5. Don't read in bed or slouch in a low chair with most of the weight of your upper torso on the back of your neck; neither should you read while lying on your stomach with your head extended backward.

6. Do not sleep on thick, hard pillows. A cervical pillow that fits the curve of your neck may be helpful. It is available from most physical therapists or orthopaedic surgeons. Avoid sleeping on your stomach.

7. Above all, adjust the mechanics of placing yourself in relation to what you are doing. This might mean using a stepladder for work done above your normal eye level, such as painting. It might call for a cushion in your car to keep your head above the level of your steering wheel. It almost always means having a desk chair that can be lowered so that you can comfortably keep your eyes on your desk work without neck strain.

"If despite these natural remedies you get a pain in the neck which does not respond to home treatment, consult your doctor. If you feel numbness or weakness in your hands, arms or legs, see your physician promptly," says the California Medical Association.[104]

Think of your head as a ten-pound bowling ball, with only tensed, tiny muscles in the back of your neck to stop it from falling forward. Eventually the fatigue and stress is too much and will cause a kink in your neck and pain. With the use of ongoing exercise, you can develop a stronger musculoskeletal system to resist distress and feel healthfully light-headed and youthfully flexible!

STRESS AND TENSION

Symptoms

Feelings of anxiety, constant fatigue, grinding teeth, trembling, profuse sweating, appetite disorders, irregularity or diarrhea, headaches, hyperactivity, indigestion, insomnia, various pains and aches, nervousness, skin problems, temperamental behavior, pounding heart, bulging eyes, unnatural breathing patterns.

Natural Remedies

Erwin DiCyan, Ph.D., noted psychotherapist of Brooklyn, New York cautions, "Stress can lead to life-threatening illnesses such as heart attacks, glandular upset, blood pressure disturbances. A feeling of anger worsens the stressful situation. You need to change your attitude so that you do not succumb to tensions. For example, if you believe the world is against you, then you become hostile and this leads to self-induced stress. Do not keep bringing up past hurts. Seek love and guidance. A great stress remedy: give love while you receive it! Be calm in the face of difficulty: a soft answer surely does turn away wrath! And finally, put yourself into the other person's position—ask yourself how you would feel if someone were to act against you. This approach adjusts your attitude. The best remedy of all: laugh at yourself! Laugh at the stress! It is all part of the quality of being human."[105]

Nutritional Remedies to Erase Stress. How your body and mind handle stress is directly related to nutritional status. You can cope with day-to-day stress if you are properly nourished. Some nutrients appear to be more beneficial as stress-shields:

B-complex Vitamins. These vitamins help your nervous system function optimally, they ease nerve stress, and protect against depression and irritability.

Vitamin C. Needed to meet the challenges of daily stress. This vitamin helps reduce the hurtful effects of stress hormones and boosts the body's ability to adequately handle stress response.

Calcium. Soothes the nervous system, helps regulate your heartbeat, stabilizes your pulse, insulates your senses against the shocks of abrasive stress.

Magnesium. Needed in your tissues to meet the challenges of stress. Gives you a feeling of calmness in the face of strife.

Fitness: Protection Against Stress. "The ability to handle stress is as important as, if not more important than, native managerial ability in rising to the top and functioning effectively once there," says James Rippe, M.D., Director of the Exercise Physiology and Nutrition Laboratory at the University of Massachusetts Medical School, Boston.

Dr. Rippe believes that exercise is effective against stress because it produces beta-endorphins, the powerful, morphine-like substances that are linked to feelings of well-being. He points out that being fit can help in situations where exercise is impossible. Conditioned bodies adapt more efficiently than others to stress, pumping out less adrenaline and thereby limiting the degree to which your heartbeat increases. "Moreover, when you're in good shape, your body will release endorphins at stressful times—just when you need them most."[106]

Four Quick Ways to Reduce Stress. Try these remedies if you feel yourself tightening up with stress.

1. Close your eyes and draw ten deep, cleansing breaths. Picture yourself surrounded by soothing things.
2. Shower with warm to cool water, as opposed to hot. Direct heat will dry your skin and leave you more apt to feel drowsy than revitalized.
3. Take a nice long bath (water can be a little warmer here). Place cucumber slices or moistened tea bags over eye area. Then just sit back and relax.
4. Smile more, frown less. Smiling places less stress on your skin. Frowning will create more lines and uses more energy.

Belly Breathing Soothes Stress. Under stress, your pulse races, and you breathe rapidly. Correct yourself at once. Force yourself to breathe slowly. Let your abdomen expand as you inhale and deflate as you exhale. Do this for five minutes, and you will defeat nervousness and anxiety.

Become Assertive Instead of Aggressive. If someone's behavior is irritating, calmly explain what is bothering you and why you would like them to stop. Do not attack them personally. And . . . learn the power of forgiveness. Compassion is the strongest natural remedy for angry stress.

STOMACH ACHE OR CRAMPS

Symptoms

Also called cramps or an upset stomach, stomach ache causes a feeling of fullness or discomfort in the stomach or lower chest area, accompanied by belching or burning sensations.

Natural Remedies

Make friends with your stomach with better living methods to ease and prevent a hurtful upset. Follow this set of natural remedies and enjoy a healthier digestive system.

1. *Eat meals slowly. Chew your food thoroughly.* The smaller the food particles are, the more surface they present to digestive juices for easier digestion. Chewing stimulates more saliva secretion, which lubricates and has a solvent action on food that improves taste.

2. *Limit Foods that Are Too Spicy.* While seasoning enhances the taste and enjoyment of food, it should be used in moderation. Too much seasoning can irritate your stomach's lining.

3. *Avoid Foods with a High Fat Content.* If food has a high concentration of fat, or has been fried in fat, the reaction in the stomach is the same as eating too fast. Just as your digestive system can handle only so much food at one time, so, too, can it break down only so much fat at one time. When you swallow fatty foods, signals are sent to your liver and gallbladder to secrete bile, which is needed to break down fat. If too much fat is consumed, too much bile is secreted, and your stomach lining becomes irritated.

4. *Avoid Drinking Water with Your Meals.* Far better to do your drinking two hours before or two hours after meals. Food should not be waterlogged, which may cause distress.

5. *Alcohol Can Upset Your Stomach.* Alcohol irritates your digestive system. It can cause inflammation of the mucous membrane surface of the stomach lining. This can bring on a feeling of nausea and upset stomach. **CAUTION:** Alcohol stimulates secretion of gastric acid. It delays the process that allows acid to leave your stomach. This causes a backup of acid. Over a period of time, this excess acid irritates and damages the lining of the stomach.

6. *Tobacco Can Upset Your Stomach.* Tar and smoke irritants stimulate the secretion of saliva as they are inhaled into the body. An excess of saliva irritates the stomach lining. Avoid smoking . . . your own and inhaling sidestream smoke from others, too!

7. *Be Calm or Your Stomach Becomes Upset.* Strain from nervousness or tension forces your stomach to release excessive amounts of digestive juices (acid). If there is no food present to break

down, these acids irritate your stomach lining. If you are under constant strain and upset stomach recurs frequently, then too much acid can actually eat away a part of your stomach lining, causing a gastric ulcer.

8. *Be Careful About Bicarbonate Soda.* It may be quick-acting, but its antacid effect is short-lived. Frequent or excessive use may produce increased blood alkalinity—which, ironically, may lead to the same symptoms for which the bicarbonate was taken.

How to Settle an Upset Stomach. Bedrest, with nothing by mouth until the feelings of nausea disappear. Then light fluids (herbal tea, strained broth, cereal), and when these are well tolerated, gradual addition of other foods.

SUNBURN

Symptoms

Overexposure to the sun leads to premature aging, a rough, leathery texture, freckle-like spots of brown pigmentation, discoloration, burning sensation, peeling. The degree of redness may range from mild to severe.

Natural Remedies

Here is a set of simple guidelines prepared by the Skin Cancer Foundation, to help protect you from the damaging rays of the sun.

1. **Minimize sun exposure** during the hours of 10 A.M. to 2 P.M. (11 A.M. to 3 P.M. daylight saving time) when the sun is strongest. Try to plan your outdoor activities for the early morning or late afternoon.

2. **Wear a hat,** long-sleeved shirts and long pants when out in the sun. Choose tightly-woven materials for greater protection from the sun's rays.

3. **Apply a sunscreen** before every exposure to the sun, and reapply frequently and liberally, at least every two hours, as long as you stay in the sun. The sunscreen should always be reapplied after swimming or perspiring heavily, since products differ in

their degrees of water resistance. We recommend sunscreens with an SPF (sun protection factor) of 15 or more printed on the label.*

4. **Use a sunscreen** during high altitude activities such as mountain climbing and skiing. At high altitudes, where there is less atmosphere to absorb the sun's rays, your risk of burning is greater. The sun also is stronger near the equator where the sun's rays strike the earth most directly.

5. **Don't forget to use your sunscreen** on overcast days. The sun's rays are as damaging to your skin on cloudy, hazy days as they are on sunny days.

6. **Individuals at high risk for skin cancer** (outdoor workers, fair-skinned individuals, and persons who have already had skin cancer) should apply sunscreens daily.

7. **Photosensitivity**—an increased sensitivity to sun exposure—is a possible side effect of certain medications, drugs and cosmetics, and of birth control pills. Consult your physician or pharmacist before going out in the sun if you're using any such products. You may need to take extra precautions.

8. **If you develop an allergic reaction** to your sunscreen, change sunscreens. One of the many products on the market today should be right for you.

9. **Beware of reflective surfaces!** Sand, snow, concrete and water can reflect more than half the sun's rays onto your skin. Sitting in the shade does not guarantee protection from sunburn.

10. **Avoid tanning parlors.** The UV light emitted by tanning booths causes sunburn and premature aging, and increases your risk of developing skin cancer.

11. **Keep young infants out of the sun.** Begin using sunscreens on children at six months of age, and then allow sun exposure with moderation.

12. **Teach children sun protection early.** Sun damage occurs with each unprotected sun exposure and accumulates over the course of a lifetime.[108]

Cool Off the Heat. If you have a burn, try these cooling compresses. (You could also aim a fan on the sunburned region to make it feel cooler.)

---

* The Skin Cancer Foundation grants its Seal of Recommendation to sunscreen products of SPF 15 or greater and sun protection devices which meet the Foundation's criteria as "aids in the prevention of sun-induced damage to the skin."

Cold Water. Dip a clean cloth in plain water or ice cold water. Place it over the burned area. Repeat whenever the cloth warms. Apply a few times throughout the day.

Milk Cooler. Dip a clean cloth in a mixture of one cup skim milk with four cups of ice water. Place the cloth over the hurt area. Repeat when the cloth warms. Apply several times during the day. The milk protein is said to be most soothing.

Oatmeal Compress. Wrap ordinary dry oatmeal in gauze or cheese-cloth. Run cool water through it. Save the water in a bowl. Discard the oatmeal. Soak clean cloth in this oatmeal water and apply to the hurt area. Repeat every few hours.

Witch Hazel. An old-time remedy, it works! Dip cotton balls into witch hazel and gently—that's gently!—stroke on the burned area.

Yogurt Is Cooling. Apply plain yogurt to the burned area for quick cooling. Rinse off in a cool shower and gently pat dry.

Baking Soda Bath. Dissolve some baking soda in lukewarm bath-water and enjoy a cooling-healing soak. Instead of towel drying, let the solution dry on your skin.

Drink Lots of Water. Your body and skin have become dehydrated, so drink lots of plain water throughout the day for more moisture.

Finally, keep soap use to a minimum. It can irritate your burned skin. For cleanliness, use a mild soap and splash off thoroughly. Avoid soapy water . . . keep away from bubble baths. And . . . use more sun-sense the next time!

T

THYROID GLAND

Symptoms

A butterfly-shaped gland, situated in the back of the neck, it releases thyroxin, an iodine-containing hormone that is essential for normal metabolic processes and mental and physical development.

An overactive thyroid causes excessive sweating, weight loss and increased appetite, tiredness, and nervousness. There may be a swollen neck (goiter), muscle weakness, bulging eyes, and bone loss, predisposing to osteoporosis.

An underactive thyroid is sluggish and causes poor toleration to cold, lack of energy, dry, rough skin, water retention, lethargy, slow speech, and goiter.

Natural Remedies

To help improve the balance of the thyroid, nutritional remedies are available for each of the extremes.

Overactive Thyroid. Increase the quantity of fluids you consume and aim for about three quarts per day. Boost intake of calcium through non-fat dairy products and supervised supplement. For bulging eyes, cut down consumption of salt to shrink the swelling behind the eyes. Control intake of sharply spiced foods and those containing caffeine because they increase frequency of bowel movements. Because an overactive thyroid increases the metabolic rate, you will need more B-complex and C vitamins, along with minerals. Avoid alcohol because it blocks the liver from making glucose; if glucose levels drop below normal, you may be light-headed or feel faint.

Underactive Thyroid. Control food intake because you have a sluggish metabolism and therefore need fewer calories. Because of this slowdown, you need to include more roughage or fiber to protect against constipation. You need at least 18 milligrams of iron and 400 micrograms of folic acid daily. Food sources include apples, green beans, lean beef, brewer's yeast, broccoli, liver (high in cholesterol), orange juice, poultry, amaranth grains, dried figs, blackstrap molasses, cooked peas, and soybean curd. Iodine is readily available in such foods as seafood, milk, meat, kelp, seaweed. Vitamin A is important because you have a lowered ability to convert beta-carotene, the form of this nutrient found in plant foods. You may develop a sallow skin and a vitamin A deficiency. Vitamin A is found in eggs, beef liver, yogurt, and whole milk. (Careful, these foods are also high in cholesterol and fat.)

A healthy thyroid helps build a healthy body and mind . . . and with nutritional remedies, you can achieve this goal!

TRAVELER'S DIARRHEA

Symptoms

So, you're going on a trip. The reservations are made, the money paid, your bags packed. You're prepared for every contingency—or are you? What about the most important aspect of any travel plan—your health! Nothing can ruin a costly foreign vacation or business trip more quickly than diarrhea and its familiar abdominal cramps. "Montezuma's revenge," "turista," and "Tut's tummy" are among the many nicknames given this unpleasant ailment.

Almost always the problem is due to inadequate sanitation. Contaminated food and water contain bacteria that attach themselves to the lining of your small intestine and release a toxin that causes diarrhea and cramps. The germ most often responsible is known as enterotoxigenic *E. coli*. Entero means intestine. Toxigenic means to produce a toxin, or poison, and *E. coli* is the scientific name of the bacterium.

Traveler's diarrhea is common in many parts of the world, particularly in the developing countries. High-risk areas include Latin America, Africa, the Middle East and Asia, but you also need to be careful in much of southern Europe and some Caribbean islands. *Note:* If you stay two weeks in some of these places, your chance of getting ill goes up 50 percent, and this refers to an illness lasting an average of five days, which could confine you to bed.

Natural Remedies

A set of guidelines is offered by Charles Ericsson, M.D., Associate Professor of Microbiology and Infectious Diseases, and expert on travelers' diarrhea, at the University of Texas in Austin. It should help you prevent the disorder.

1. Prevention begins en route. While you're on the plane, exercise every hour by stretching or walking the aisle. Eat lightly. Drink plenty of juice. **CAREFUL**: Carbonated beverages can cause stomach upsets at high altitudes.

2. When you arrive, watch what you drink. Select distilled bottled water. Don't accept anything someone wants to palm off on you. Experienced travelers take a heating coil and boil the water, to be sure.

3. On land, carbonated beverages are ideal, because the same process that creates the fizz helps knock out bugs.

4. Alcohol is **not** ideal unless the ice cubes chilling it are made from purified water. Many tourists are under the impression that alcohol kills organisms. We tried it in the lab and it works—but it takes hours.

5. Food, which causes 90 percent of the diarrhea problem, should only be eaten steaming hot. No matter how good it looks, pass up those homemade sauces that sit on the table—unless they come out of a bottle with a brand name, and you see the sealed bottle opened in front of you.

6. Eat only fruit that you peel yourself. Dry foods like bread are safe, but salads, uncooked vegetables, and dairy products are on the forbidden list. *Note*: Pasteurized dairy products should be safe from some bacteria. Milk powder reconstituted with boiled water is preferable.

7. Be careful *where* you eat. Don't go to a dive just because it looks like a lot of fun. Go to major, well-traveled restaurants that are in the tourist guides, or ask the advice of local friends.[109]

Hints, Tips, Suggestions. Remember that you are safer with fruits (bananas, melons, citrus) that can be eaten raw, fruits that grow on trees and can be peeled, such as apples. Use bottled water to brush your teeth. In the tropics, fresh milk should be boiled before use or, alternatively, mix powdered milk with boiled water. If you cannot resist native raw fish delicacies, make sure the fish are salt water, not fresh water, varieties. Drink boiled water, hot beverages, bottled carbonated water, and bottled or canned drinks from their original containers.

Treating Diarrhea. A helpful remedy is recommended by the U.S. Public Health Service for helping overcome traveler's diarrhea:
You need two separate glasses.

Glass Number One: Eight ounces orange, apple or other fruit juice; ½ teaspoon honey; one pinch table salt.

Glass Number Two: Eight ounces boiled or carbonated water; ¼ teaspoon baking soda (sodium bicarbonate).

Remedy: Drink alternately from each glass until thirst is quenched. Supplement as desired with carbonated beverages, water or tea made with boiled or carbonated water. Avoid solid food or milk until recovery occurs.[110]

Quick Remedy for Diarrhea. A folk remedy suggests cooking apple peels and drinking the liquid. It is rich in pectin, used for making jelly, and helpful in halting diarrhea.

Replace Those Lost Minerals. Severe diarrhea causes large losses of water and electrolytes needed for normal functioning of body tissues. *To Replace:* drink combinations of fruit juice (for potassium), a pinch of salt (for sodium and chloride), and honey (for glucose and fructose), and you will replace lost electrolytes. As the diarrhea subsides, reintroduce solid foods . . . slowly. CAREFUL: After a bout with traveler's diarrhea, your intestinal walls are severely irritated. Do not worsen by eating high-fiber foods. Instead, try soft, easily digestible foods for the first few days.

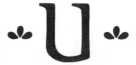

ULCERS

Symptoms

An ulcer is a painful hole in the lining of the stomach, which goes through the mucous membrane or top layer of the stomach lining, through the next thin layer of muscle, called the muscularis mucosa, and into the fibrous lining known as the sub-mucosa. The basic ulcers include: *duodenal ulcers*, which exist in the form of a broken mucous membrane and possibly a sore, which bleeds and causes some danger of perforating the intestinal wall; *gastric ulcers*, which affect the stomach; *peptic ulcers*, which occur in the lower end of the esophagus, in the stomach, usually along the lesser curvature or in the duodenum, the first part of the small intestines connecting with the lower opening of the stomach and extending to the remainder of the small intestine. Symptoms include discomfort and pain . . . pain . . . pain .

Natural Remedies

Let's separate fact from fiction about ulcer care. Jon I. Isenberg, M.D., Professor of Medicine at The University of California, San Diego points out, "Thinking in terms of what you *can* do, rather than what you *cannot* do, may enhance the ability to cope with flare-ups." The guidelines consist of seven basic do's and don't:

1. *Smoking.* "I urge you to stop smoking. There is much evidence it is associated with peptic ulcer formation. There is slower healing, and smokers have more complications and are more likely to require surgical treatment than non-smokers," says Dr. Isenberg.

2. *Aspirin.* "It damages the lining of the stomach and can cause ulcers. Eliminate all self-medication with products containing aspirin. Enteric-coated aspirin causes less damage from direct irritation, but after absorption may still have harmful systemic effects."

3. *Non-steroidal Anti-inflammatory Drugs.* "Used to treat arthritis, it may also damage the lining of the stomach, cause erosions and ulcers and may worsen ulcer disease. In this event, your

physician can usually change medication schedules or reduce individual doses to overcome the problem. Products containing acetaminophen have not been found to be harmful to patients with peptic ulcer."

4. *Sodium Bicarbonate*. "It is a potent neutralizer of acid. If used repetitively, it delivers an overload of sodium. Your body then retains water, may increase blood pressure, or exacerbate heart disease. **DANGER:** Sodium bicarbonate with milk, as used by many who have chronic stomach pain can cause the milk-alkali syndrome. This has a serious array of symptoms including raising blood calcium, causing calcium-containing kidney stones, and kidney failure. The repetitive use of baking soda is dangerous for peptic ulcer."

5. *Alcohol*. "Chronic use of alcohol can cause gastritis that can mimic ulcer symptoms."

6. *Food*. Dr. Isenberg emphasizes, "Ulcer patients should learn to challenge myths about foods." He gives these tips:

- Meat is **not** ulcerogenic. Vegetarians have the same incidence of peptic ulcer disease as non-vegetarians.

- Spicy foods do **not** cause or aggravate ulcers. Mexican-Americans, who consume great quantities of red-hot peppers, for example, are no more prone to peptic ulcer disease than any other ethnic or cultural group.

- Milk is **not** a substitute for medical treatment. While milk does temporarily relieve the pain of peptic ulcers by neutralizing acid, it is a potent stimulant of acid production and therefore, perpetuates the need for further neutralizing.

- Many ulcer patients claim one food or another exacerbates their pain. To them I would say, avoid *anything* that causes you distress, so long as you remain on a balanced diet. I might add, however, that avoiding particular foods will not in itself enhance ulcer healing.

- Maintain a normal, three-meals-a-day schedule. Frequent small meals continuously stimulate the stomach to produce acid and pepsin (enzyme found in gastric juice, believed to contribute to peptic ulcer formation). Having a snack at bedtime may even cause sleep-disrupting pain.

7. *Stress*. "There is no convincing evidence that stress causes ulcers. Quantitation of stress is difficult and the causes of stress varies from person to person. Avoiding fear or anxiety-provoking stress whenever possible, is a good thing for ulcer patients. But the same is surely true for everybody else as well. I know of absolutely

no reason to tell ulcer patients to avoid excitement or exhilarating stress. Stress for one person may be tranquility for others. Many people thrive on it. Many others would give a lot—perhaps even risk an ulcer—to experience it."[111]

Is There an "Ulcer Personality"? "No such stereotyped personality seems to exist," notes Seymour M. Sabesin, M.D., Professor of Medicine, University of Tennessee Center of Health Sciences, in Memphis. The ailment "occurs in those who seem easygoing just as frequently as in the tense, hard-driving person. The high-powered executive in a competitive business situation is no more prone to developing ulcers than someone in a less competitive situation."[112]

Yet it would make good sense to shield yourself from stressful situations. Being high-strung, a perfectionist, subjected to unrelieved tension may well create a susceptibility to ulcers (among other ailments), so it would be wise to practice relaxation techniques. When you relax your mind, you relax your body. And finally, be aware of your own reactions. If anything causes unrest, keep away from it . . . and your ulcer will heal all the better.

URINARY TRACT INFECTION

Symptoms

Each year, one in five women experience the discomforts of a urinary tract infection (UTI), characterized by a frequent and urgent need to urinate, a sharp, burning sensation, and, often, the presence of blood in the urine. Some may notice an ache in the area of the bladder or in the lower back in the area of the kidneys. Fever is an important symptom of UTI, especially if it occurs at the same time as some of the other symptoms. The bacteria most often responsible for the infection are called *E-coli*. They usually originate in the bowel, travel across the perineum (the area between the anus and the vagina) and then up the urethra to the bladder. Some women are more prone to UTIs, because either their defense mechanisms are inadequate, or the bacteria are of a particularly virulent strain and can attach themselves to mucosal surfaces and invade the urinary tract. They are most common in sexually active women but they can affect men and women of all ages. **CAUTION:** Postmenopausal women are at increased risk for UTI. The decreased level of estrogen affects the functioning of the bladder and urethra. The tissue becomes thinner and more vulnerable to infection when the ovaries stop working.

Natural Remedies

To ease symptoms and help clear up UTI, some better self-care will be useful. These include:

Drink More Liquids. Especially water. It helps flush bacteria out of the urinary tract. CAREFUL: The longer the bacteria stays in your bladder, the more it will multiply. *E. coli* doubles its amount about every 20 minutes—more bacteria means more pain. Therefore, to fight the burning, drink fluids to flush out the inflammation-causing bacteria. (*Quick Test*: If your urine is clear, you are drinking enough water. If it is dark, you are not!)

What About Cranberry Juice? It contains quinolic acid, which changes into hippuric acid in the liver. The acidic reaction is believed to be beneficial in defusing the infection. Several glasses of cranberry juice daily may do the trick.

Vitamin C To the Rescue. To help kill the infection, you need to acidify your urine. About 1,000 milligrams taken throughout the day will help create this reaction that will interfere with runaway bacterial growth. (*Note*: Some prescribed antibiotics for UTI do not work well in acidic urine; discuss your use of vitamin C with your doctor so that potencies meet with medical approval.)

Ease Discomfort With Warm Bath. A comfortably warm bath tends to ease pain, particularly the inflammation. About 20 minutes will cool off the hurt.

Observe Personal Hygiene. Wear cotton underwear to keep you dry. Avoid tight garments that block ventilation. After a bathroom trip, wipe from front to back to prevent infection from recurring. Wiping the wrong way can send bacteria into your system. Remember, you need to move bacteria *away* from your openings, not toward them! And be sure to bathe often to remove bacteria from the perineal region. And . . . void completely before and after intercourse . . . finishing with a glass of water.

CASE HISTORY—*Cools Off "Burning Urine" with Home Remedies*

A shock went through Helen P. when she passed urine. The burning was agonizing. There were spasms in the small of her back that sent her into a panic. Were her kidneys failing? She wisely sought help from her gynecologist, who diagnosed it as a urinary tract infection. She was already in her menopause which made her more susceptible to the bacterial invasion. Helen P. was told to drink at least six glasses of fresh water daily. She was also told to add at least two glasses of cranberry juice to her program and a 1,000 milligram supplement of vitamin C daily. She was instructed on how to observe personal hygiene. Within seven days, she no longer screamed when she voided. The burning had cooled off. In three more weeks, diagnostic tests showed she had defeated the *E-coli* bacteria . . . they had diminished . . . and Helen P. could live normally again!

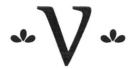

VAGINITIS

Symptoms

Any infection or inflammation of the vagina may be referred to as vaginitis. The cause may be a fungus, bacteria, virus or other organism. Vaginitis may occur with or without sexual contact. These conditions nearly always result in extreme discomfort such as severe itching, pain on urinating or in the pelvis. There may be redness, irritation, and inflammation, as well as unusual or unpleasant odors and discharges. A weakness in your immune system may be a major cause of lowered resistance—from stress, malnutrition, lack of sleep, or another infection elsewhere in the body.

Other Causes of Vaginitis. The vaginal area may have an adverse reaction to chemicals such as those used in feminine hygiene sprays or bubble baths. If injury to the vaginal walls occurs (for example, from improper tampon use), or if the outside organs are irritated by tight clothing or fabrics that don't "breathe," then redness, swelling, and discharge can result. Synthetic hormones (such as birth control pills) can also alter the hormonal balance of the vagina and cause symptoms. In postmenopausal women, the vaginal tissues are no longer stimulated by the female hormone estrogen, from the ovaries. Tissue thins and becomes dry. The vagina is more prone to injury and can more easily become irritated.

Natural Remedies

If you have recurrent vaginitis, try some of these natural remedies.

Yogurt. A dairy product that has been fermented with the bacteria culture *Lactobacillus acidophilus.* This bacteria is most effective in protecting the body from outside pathogens. Try a yogurt douche, which has long been a common folk healer for vaginal tract infections.
Try any of these helpful remedies to ease vaginitis:
—Avoid spreading bacteria from the rectum to the vagina. After a bowel movement, wipe from front to back, away from the vagina.
—Clean your vulva thoroughly. Keep as dry as possible.

—Avoid irritating substances—harsh soaps or detergents, feminine hygiene sprays, perfumed toilet paper, perfumed tampons.

—Avoid using tampons solely throughout your entire menstrual period.

—Thoroughly clean diaphragms and spermicide applicators.

—Avoid tight jeans, panties or panty hose without a cotton crotch, or other clothing that can trap moisture.

—Keep the vulva as dry as possible. The infection spreads in moisture and heat. This means careful drying after a bath or shower, wearing cotton (rather than nylon or other synthetic) underpants. Change from bathing suits soon after swimming. Clothing that comes in contact with your vulva should be washed between wearing.

—Except for a yogurt douche, avoid other douches, which can wash away some vital organisms.

—Cut down on coffee, alcohol, sugar, and refined carbohydrates. Diets high in sugars can radically change the normal pH—acid-alkaline balance—of the vagina.

—Do alert your sexual partner. He, too, may be infected and, in many instances, should also be treated. This will help avoid reinfection.

VARICOSE VEINS

Symptoms

Varicose veins are veins that have become swollen or twisted, either because of a weakness in the vein wall, or a faulty valve somewhere in the vein itself. For either of these situations, aching legs, with bulging bumps and discolored skin, are evidence of the condition. It is also called venous insufficiency. There are prominently visible veins. Or there may be spider veins or spider bursts, those dilated tiny veins lying within the layers of the skin. Calf muscle cramps, occurring especially at night, are often recurring symptoms. So is itching or a burning sensation over a prominent varicosity.

Why does it happen? Considering that the veins of your leg support a column of blood of considerable height, it is not surprising that dilated and varicose veins are common. With every step, a column of blood several feet high pounds the veins of the legs like a battering ram. The repeated impacts encourage phlebitis (inflammation of the vein wall). Moreover, if clots or crusts are present in the veins (they usually stick to the inner surface), the impact may release them into the bloodstream and cause them to be swept into the heart and lungs, causing thrombophlebitis.

Other causes include pregnancy, chronic constipation (increased pressure on the veins), low fiber diet, obesity, prolonged sitting or standing.

Natural Remedies

Here are some recommendations considered helpful for those with this ailment:

1. When on a long plane or train trip, get up and walk around every half hour. Or on a long auto trip, stop every so often, and get out to stretch your legs.
2. While reading or watching television, elevate your feet. Rest your legs on a chair or stool. The practice of putting feet on a desk is helpful.
3. Exercise helps the general circulation. Walking is especially beneficial because the movements of leg muscles help push the blood upward. **TIP:** Swimming or walking in deep water does much the same thing; the great pressure of the water against the legs helps move the blood up the veins.
4. Sleeping with feet raised slightly above the level of the heart helps blood flow away from the ankle. (This is not advisable for some people. Check with your health practitioner.) If you have serious trouble with varicose veins, raise your bed by placing 6-inch-high blocks under the bedposts at the foot. This gives better support than simply raising the mattress.
5. For those confined to bed, movement of feet or legs should be encouraged, to help the circulation.
6. Round garters should never be worn. They cut off the venous circulation, thus raising pressure in the veins and increasing the risk of varicosities.
7. Elastic girdles should not be worn continuously—especially when you will be seated for a long time, such as at a desk, or during a plane, train or auto trip. They bunch up and hamper the return flow of blood. This increases the pressure of the blood in the veins and worsens varicosities.
8. Pregnant patients may find it helpful to wear elastic stockings and to lie down occasionally during the day. Getting up soon after delivery is also important.
9. If elastic stockings are prescribed, they should be worn continuously, except in bed.

10. Many women minimize the appearance of elastic stockings by wearing them underneath ordinary stockings in fashionable shades.

11. Never cross your legs—constant pressure will compress the veins. Again, put your feet up whenever possible.

12. Do not stand in one place for a long time. This only exacerbates the blood's draining back into the veins.

13. Avoid constricting garments. Wear pantyhose with light support. Remember—moderate pressure on the veins is better.

14. Periodically rise up on your toes should you be stuck in one spot for long. Keep wriggling your toes.

15. Watch your weight. Obesity means more pressure on your legs, one reason why pregnant women often develop the ailment. Keep your weight down, and you'll have fewer problems with bulging veins.

VIRUSES

Symptoms

A virus is a submicroscopic microbe, which causes infectious disease. It can reproduce only in living cells. Every time a microbe slips into your body through the slightest cut or sore, it represents a threat to your health. Your immune system is that much weaker. The virus penetrates the cell and causes havoc. The last time you had a cold, you could blame it on this entity, the virus. Many illnesses, major and minor, are caused by viral infections: measles, mumps, polio, hepatitis, rabies, certain pneumonias, some cancers and, of course, flu and some intestinal upsets. Viruses are also believed to trigger AIDS. And the genital herpes simplex virus has disrupted the personal lives of millions of people. In addition, viruses may play a role in such illnesses as multiple sclerosis, diabetes, even Alzheimer's disease. To help resist the impact of viral infections, your goal is to boost your immune response.

Natural Remedies

"Moderation remains the key to a health-promoting diet and a healthy immune system," says Ranjit J. Chandra, M.D., pediatrician and immunologist at the Memorial University of Newfoundland, who offers this set of immune-boosting, virus-fighting remedies:

Vitamin A—helps build immunity to infection. Found in dark-green and deep-yellow fruits and vegetables.

Vitamin B₆—needed to boost cellular and hormone-regulated immunity. Found in whole grains and greens.

Folic Acid—needed for cell division and immune response. Found in organ meats and most greens.

Zinc—helps in the maturation of immunological cells, enhancing the immune response. Found in meat, eggs, poultry, and seafood.

Selenium—needed for the formation of antibodies and enzymes that participate in immunity. Found in whole grain cereals, seafood, meat, poultry, milk, garlic, and egg yolk (which is high in cholesterol).

Omega-3 Fatty Acids—believed to be useful in helping to stop the spread of cancer cells; useful in accelerating the vigorous activity of white blood cells, which protect against illness and viral invaders.

Dr. Chandra sees nutrition as a promising remedy to help build a strong fortress against viral diseases.[113]

Vitamin C Stimulates Immune Response. This virus-buster works in your body as a scavenger, picking up all sorts of debris—cleansing your body of the hurtful invaders. Vitamin C strengthens your body's defense against invasion, boosting production of T-lymphocytes, which do battle with the viruses and help wash them out of your system.

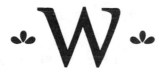

WARTS

Symptoms

Warts are growths on the skin caused by viruses. They are contagious, unsightly, and frequently painful. They come in many sizes and shapes and can turn up on different parts of the body. The so-called common wart is a raised, rough, grayish-looking, painless growth. Size varies from a pinhead to a large mass. They are usually found on the fingers, hands, and soles of the feet.

Natural Remedies

Jerome Z. Litt, M.D., renowned dermatologist of Case Western University of Medicine, Cleveland, Ohio tells us, "Some doctors recommend that the best way to manage warts is to let them manage themselves. If left untreated, many warts will disappear by themselves in about two years. This seems to be the natural history of warts. But warty people may not want to wait for any spontaneous cure, so they seek medical advice." He offers these remedies:

Stubborn Warts Around and Under Fingernails. Completely wrap the wart with four layers of plain adhesive. Don't wrap too tightly! Leave on for 6½ days. Remove for half a day. Repeat the entire procedure (6½ days on, ½ day off). After three or four weeks, the wart "gets tired" and disappears, leaving no scar.

Small, Flat Warts, on Face and Backs of Hands. Apply castor oil twice daily, using a cotton-tipped applicator.[114]

Vitamin C Remedy. A folk healer calls for crushing several vitamin C tablets, making a paste with water, covering with a bandage. It is believed that the high acidity of the vitamin may kill the wart-causing virus and bring about relief.

Hints, Tips, Suggestions The wart-causing virus can be picked up in the air or via moisture, as you would pick up any viral infection. To lessen your vulnerability, always wear plastic thong sandals around

271

swimming pools and public locker rooms. (Tiny cracks or cuts in your feet could be invaded by the virus.) Avoid moisture by changing shoes frequently, letting your shoes dry out between wearings. Did you suddenly see a wart? Don't touch! Any slight scratch on your finger and the virus could spread and penetrate! For some, warts can be "imagined" away via the power of suggestion. Visualize your warts shrinking, dissolving . . . do this about ten minutes each day over a period of time. Many have found this remedy to work. But only if you believe it at the start!

Vitamin Remedy. You will need a prescription of vitamin A acid! Apply to your wart. Cover with a tape. Let it remain for four weeks. It may well do the trick!

WRINKLES

Symptoms

Creases, folds, sags of the skin—anywhere on the body but more noticeably on the face. Although there are many rewards with age, there are some penalties . . . and the biggest ones are those unsightly wrinkles that make you look much older than you are. You may feel older, too!

Natural Remedies

Overexposure to the sun is the primary cause of aging skin. The wrinkles, the leathery and rough texture, the age spots are due to sun damage. The sun penetrates the lower skin layer, where it damages the collagen and elastin so that skin loses its elasticity and firmness. Some of the pigment-forming cells at the base of the epidermis are stimulated to produce too much pigment, so spots of hyperpigmentation (age spots, "senile freckles") appear. Old Sol can make you old before your time!

Six Steps to Avoid Wrinkles. Jerome Z. Litt, M.D., dermatologist with Case Western Reserve University of Medicine comes to the point with his wrinkle-preventing program:

1. Avoid the sun! I cannot stress this enough. In otherwise healthy people, sun exposure is the principal cause not only of wrinkles, aging skin and other degenerative changes, but of skin cancers.
2. Avoid extremes of heat and cold. Protect your face against the wind and rain and snow.

3. Wash your face with a gentle soap. Avoid excessively hot water and harsh cleansers.

4. Do not lose and gain weight, off again, on again, like a yo-yo. The constant expansion and contraction of the skin will only tire out the elastic fibers.

5. No facial exercises or isometrics. These, when overdone, can cause a breakdown of the elastic fibers and the collagen in the skin.

6. And cut down on smoking.[115]

Vitamin Cream Reverses Skin Aging. John J. Voorhees, M.D., of the University of Michigan Medical Center has had much success in using a topical form of vitamin A, available by prescription, helping to minimize the hurts done to sun-damaged skin. "With tretinoin (the generic name given to this vitamin cream), new skin cells push toward the surface and this clears the skin of dead cells and other debris. There is a fading of age spots, and a stimulation of collagen production. At the same time there is an increase in the amount of blood circulating to the skin, which now has a healthier appearance. Cell growth becomes more even."

Dr. Voorhees notes, "The cream begins to work almost immediately following application. Within a week, changes begin to occur. The activities go on for some weeks before you actually see the changes. Within a month or two, the skin takes on a rosy glow, becomes less wrinkled. It has more elasticity, less blotching and has better color."[116]

Beware of Sleep Wrinkles. They happen when you push your face into your pillow at night. Train yourself to sleep on your back. Or else, try to find some comfortable position so your face is not pressing on the pillow.

Are You Feeding Yourself a Smoother Skin? Your skin cells and tissues need lots of nutrients from fresh fruits and green leafy vegetables as well as whole grains and moderate amounts of lean meats and skim-milk dairy products. Chock full of vitamins and minerals, amino acids and trace elements are needed for a healthy skin.

Lots of Water. Your thirsty skin cells need much liquids throughout the day. Plump up your collagen with fresh water as well as succulent fruits and vegetables. Together with an external moisturizer, you will help improve the elastic quality of your skin so it springs back to a youthfully firm shape.

Wash . . . but Don't Overwash. Keeping your skin clean is important but excessive washing and scrubbing, especially with harsh soaps and very hot water will break down elastic fibers and dissolve essential oils that are needed to nourish the skin. **TIP:** Spend more time rinsing and less time washing. Do **not** let any soapy film remain on your skin or it will cause wrinkling.

Avoid a Dry Home. It can dry out your skin! A humidifier is helpful; have an assortment of plants that you water regularly. Put small pots of water on your windowsill to help introduce more skin-nourishing water in your living space.

Moisturize Your Skin . . . Easily. After washing, apply ordinary petroleum jelly or vegetable shortening (Crisco) to your face, hands, neck. Let it remain overnight. You have "locked in" the moisture from your recent washing. Do **not** slather it on. Rub it in firmly but gently. Do this every night before you go to sleep. Next morning, wipe it off with a non-drying, alcohol-free lotion. You will be moisturizing your skin and working miracles in helping to prevent wrinkles and minimizing any that have appeared.

FOOTNOTES

1. Fulton, Jr., James E., M.D., personal interview, March, 1991

2. Pochi, Peter E., M.D., personal interview, February, 1991

3. Litt, Jerome Z., M.D., *Your Skin: From Acne to Zitts*, Dembner Books, 1989, pp. 39–46 and pp. 160–209.

4. Soltanoff, Jack, Dr., personal interview, December, 1990

5. Winick, Myron, M.D., personal interview, October, 1990

6. Andrassy, Richard J., M.D., personal interview, November, 1990

7. Chandra, R., M.D., *Food Technology*, 39:91–93, 1985

8. Weiner, R. G., M.D., *Journal of the American Medical Association, Vol. 252*, p. 1409, September, 1984

9. Rodriguez, Kassandra, M.D., personal interview, October, 1990

10. Williams, Roger J., *Prevention of Alcoholism Through Nutrition*, Bantam Books, 1984, pp. 30–49

11. Leo, M. A., et al., *New England Journal of Medicine*, Vol. 307, p. 597, September, 1982

12. Dworkin, B. D., et al., *Digestive Diseases and Sciences, Vol. 30*, pp. 30–38, p. 838, September, 1985.

13. Greger, Janet, Dr., *Journal of Food Protection*, 1985

14. Garrison, Jr., Robert H., registered pharmacist, *Nutrition Desk Reference*, Keats Publishing Inc., pp. 78–79, 1990

15. *Food Chemistry*, 22:265–268, 1984

16. *Nutrition Reports*, 3:66, and 72, 1986

17. *American Journal of Clinical Nutrition*, 36:709–720, 1982

18. Adner, Marvin, M.D., Framingham Union Hospital Press Bureau, October, 1990

19. American Heart Association, *Heart Facts*, 1991, p. 8–11

20. *American Journal of Physiology*, April, 1989, pp. 105–110

21. Tyler, Varro E., Ph.D., *Hoosier Home Remedies*, Purdue University Press, pp. 30–81, 1985

22. *Annals of Internal Medicine*, April, 1987, pp. 165–178

23. *IRCS Medical Science*, Vol. 9, p. 444, 1981

24. *American Journal of Clinical Nutrition*, Vol. 41, p. 684, April, 1985

25. *American Review of Respiratory Diseases*, Vol. 127, p. 139, 1983

26. *American Review of Respiratory Diseases*, Vol. 127, p. 143, 1983

27. *Journal of the American Medical Association*, Vol. 257, p. 1076, February 27, 1987

28. Block, Barry, D.P.M., *Foot Talk*, p. 39, Arbor House, 1984

29. Sandler, Marvin, D.P.M., *Your Guide To Foot Care*, p. 69, George F. Stickley Company, 1984

30. Soltanoff, Jack, Dr., personal interview, January, 1991

31. Soltanoff, Jack, Dr., personal interview, January, 1991

32. Garrison, Jr., Robert H. (registered pharmacist) and Somer, Elizabeth, M.A., R.D., *Nutrition Desk Reference,* Keats Publishing Inc., 1990, pp. 112–140

33. *Journal of the American Medical Association*, 259:1525–1530, 1988

34. American Cancer Society, *Cancer Facts*, 1991, pp. 6–12

35. National Cancer Institute, press bureau, October, 1990

36. Boutwell, Roswell, M.D., Tricia Smith, R.N., *"Health Matters,"* University of Wisconsin Medical School, Fall, 1989, pp. 1–2

37. *Cancer Research*, Vol. 45, p. 6519, December, 1985

38. Roberts, Elizabeth H., D.P.M., *On Your Feet,* Rodale Press, pp. 72–73, 1980

39. Block, Barry, D.P.M., *Foot Talk,* pp. 35–36, Arbor House, 1984

40. Sandler, Marvin, D.P.M., *Your Guide To Foot Care*, George F. Stickley Company, 1984, pp. 18–31

41. Gubernick, Martin, M.D., press interview, November, 1990

42. Crook, William, M.D., *Yeast Connection*, Professional Books, Jackson, Tennessee, 1989, pp. 19–53

43. Crandall, Marjorie, Ph.D., *How To Prevent Yeast Infection*, Yeast Consulting Service, Torrance, California, 1990, pp. 6–13

44. Litt, Jerome Z. M.D., *Your Skin and How To Live With It,* Ballantine Books, 1986, pp. 12–39

45. Tyler, Varro, Ph.D., *The Honest Herbal*, George F. Stickley Company, 1987, pp. 4–17

46. Connor, William, M.D., press interview, August, 1990

47. Ornish, Dean, M.D., *Dr. Dean Ornish's Program For Reversing Heart Disease*, Random House, 1990, pp. 14–106

48. Ellis, John, M.D., *Southern Medical Journal*, Vol. 80, No. 7, pp. 882–884, July, 1987

49. *Journal of the American Medical Association*, May 8, 1987, pp. 187–189

50. Anderson, James W., M.D., press interview, August, 1990

51. Connor, William, M.D., press interview, September, 1990

52. Gabrielson, Ira, M.D., Medical College of Pennsylvania, Press Bureau, July, 1990

53. California Medical Association, *Health Tips*, Index #72, October, 1989

54. *American Journal of Clinical Nutrition*, April 1988, pp. 144–53

55. Williams, Sue Rodwell, R.D., Ph.D., *Handbook of Commonsense Nutrition*, C. V. Mosby Company, 1983, p. 94

56. National Institutes of Health, *Age,* 1982

57. Block, Barry, D.P.M., *Foot Talk*, p. 35, Arbor House, 1984

58. Roberts, Elizabeth, D.P.M., *On Your Feet*, Rodale Press, 1980, p. 75–90

59. Laurensen, Niels, M.D., *Listen To Your Body*, Berkeley Books, 1983, p. 463

60. DiCyan, Erwin, Ph.D., Brooklyn, New York, personal interview, December, 1990

61. Slagle, Priscilla, M.D., *"The Way Up From Down,"* UCLA Press Bureau, October, 1990

62. Litt, Jerome Z., M.D., *Your Skin: From Acne to Zitts*, Dembner Books, 1989, p. 111–139

63. Baylor College of Medicine, *Living With Allergies*, Press Bureau, October, 1990

64. American Academy of Otolaryngology, Press Bureau, November, 1990

65. Laurensen, Niels, M.D., *Listen To Your Body*, Berkeley Books, 1983, p. 166

66. Garrison, Jr., Robert H., Registered Pharmacist, *Nutrition Desk Reference*, Keats Publishing Inc., 1990, pp. 48–69

67. Tyler, Varro, Ph.D., *Hoosier Home Remedies*, Purdue University Press, 1985, pp. 19–64

68. Lesher, Jack L., Jr., M.D., Medical College of Georgia, press interview, August, 1990

69. Vickery, Donald M., and Fries, James F., *Take Care of Yourself*, Addison-Wesley Publishing Co., 1981, pp. 12–36

70. Lubitz, Arthur M., M.D., personal interview, August, 1990

71. Castell, Donald, M.D., personal interview, July, 1990

72. Atkinson, Holly, M.D., *Women and Fatigue*, Putnam Publishing Co., 1985, pp. 70–115

73. Whitehead, E. Douglas, M.D., personal interview, July, 1990

74. Chey, William Y., M.D., University of Rochester, New York, Press Bureau, September, 1989

75. Clearfield, Harris R., M.D., Hahnemann Medical College and Hospital, Press Bureau, September, 1989

76. Litt, Jerome Z., M.D., *Your Skin: From Acne to Zitts*, Dembner Books, 1989, pp. 160–209

77. Hauri, Peter, M.D., *No More Sleepless Nights*, John Wiley & Sons, 1985, pp. 34–76

78. Weiner, Michael, Ph.D., M.S., M.A. *"Weiner's Herbal,"* Stein & Day, 1980, pp. 38–94

79. Lenox Hill Hospital, New York City, Press Bureau, March, 1989

80. Cohen, Sidney, M.D., University of Pennsylvania, Press Bureau, October, 1989

81. Dement, William C., M.D., Stanford University School of Medicine, Press Bureau, September, 1990

82. Lewy, Alfred, M.D., Oregon Health Sciences University, press interview, November, 1988

83. Morgan, Brian L. G., Ph.D., *Nutrition Prescription*, Crown Publishers Inc., 1987, pp. 30–94

84. Quillin, Patrick, Ph.D., R.D., *Healing Nutrients*, Contemporary Books, 1987, pp. 46–103

85. Weil, Lowell Scott, D.P.M., Scholl College of Podiatric Medicine, Press Bureau, October, 1988

86. Fox, James M., M.D., *"Save Your Knees,"* Dell Publishing Co., 1987, pp. 30–111

87. Gray, Gary M., M.D., Stanford University Medical School, press interview, September, 1988

88. Soltanoff, Jack, Dr., West Hurley, New York, press interview, October, 1990

89. Hurwitz, Sidney, M.D., Yale University School of Medicine, interview, October, 1988

90. DiCyan, Erwin, Ph.D., Brooklyn, New York, personal interview, December, 1990

91. Lauersen, Niels, M.D., *Listen To Your Body*, Berkeley Books, 1983, pp. 39–106

92. Mowrey, Daniel B., M.D., *Lancet*, Vol. 94, March 20, 1982, p. 655.

93. DeBetz, Barbara, M.D., New York City, personal interview, December, 1990

94. Notelovitz, Morris, M.D., University of Florida College of Medicine, in Gainesville, personal interview, August, 1989

95. Shangraw, Ralph, Dr., University of Maryland, Press Bureau, December, 1988

96. Allen, Patricia, M.D., *Cycles*, Pinnacle Books, 1983, pp. 70–95

97. Lauersen, Niels H., M.D., *Pre-Menstrual Syndrome and You*, Fireside Books, New York City, 1983, pp. 81–143

98. Cohen, Jay, M.D., Postgraduate Medicine, April, 1985, pp. 111–19

99. Rudnick, Donald H., *Urology*, Vol. XXVI, No. 3, September, 1985, p. 199

100. Mills, John A., M.D., Massachusetts General Hospital, press interview, December, 1988

101. Soltanoff, Jack, Dr., West Hurley, New York, press interview, December, 1990

102. *Journal of Antimicrobial Chemotherapy*, Vol. 12, p. 489, 1983

103. Physician & Sportsmedicine, August, 1990, pp. 305–310

104. California Medical Association, *Health Tips*, Index #58, September, 1989

105. DiCyan, Erwin, Ph.D., Brooklyn, New York, personal interview, December, 1990

106. Rippe, James, M.D., *Fit For Success*, Prentice Hall, 1989, pp. 65–111

107. Skin Cancer Foundation, press interview, April, 1990

108. Skin Cancer Foundation, press interview, April, 1990

109. Ericsson, Charles, M.D., press interview, April, 1990

110. Center for Disease Control, *"Health Information for International Travel,"* U.S. Public Health Service, Atlanta, Georgia, 1988

111. Isenberg, Jon I., M.D., press interview, April, 1988

112. Sabesin, Seymour M., M.D., press interview, April, 1988

113. Chandra, Ranjit J., M.D., *Nutrition and Immunity*, Alan R. Liss, Inc., 1989, pp. 30–49

114. Litt, Jerome Z., M.D., *Your Skin: From Acne to Zitts,* Dembner Books, 1989, pp. 143–206

115. Litt, Jerome Z., M.D., *Your Skin: From Acne to Zitts*, Dembner Books, 1989, pp. 39–83

116. Voorhees, John J., M.D., press interview, November, 1989

Index